STRUCTURAL BODY WORK
and
YOGA
based on
ROLFING

Offering to

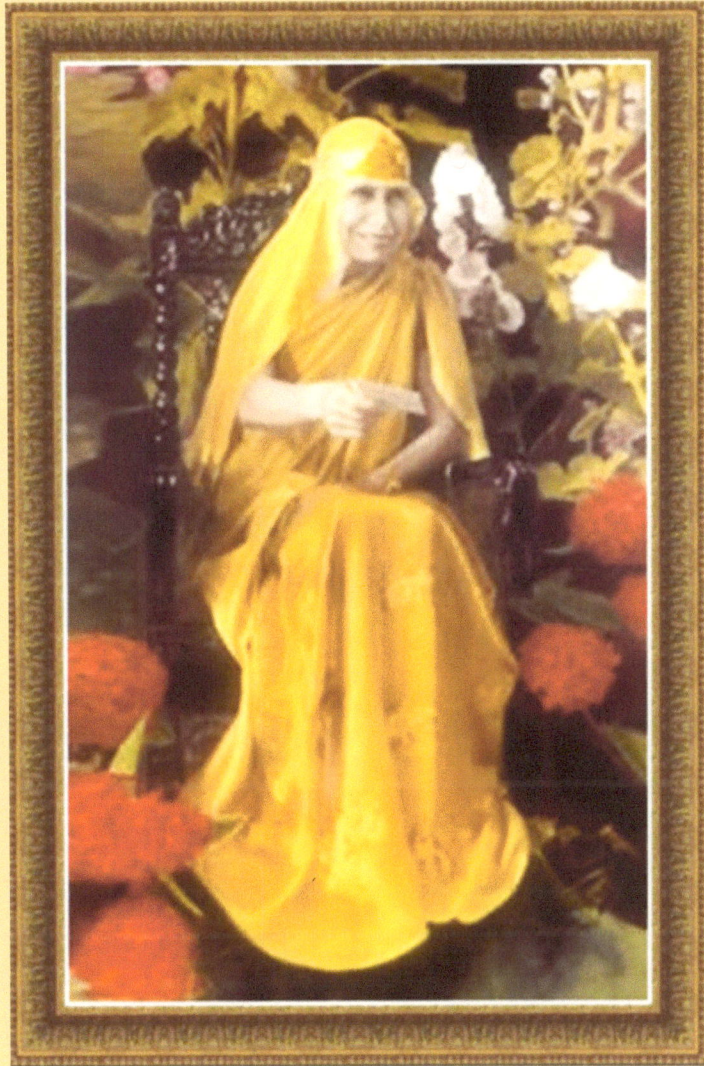

The Divine Mother

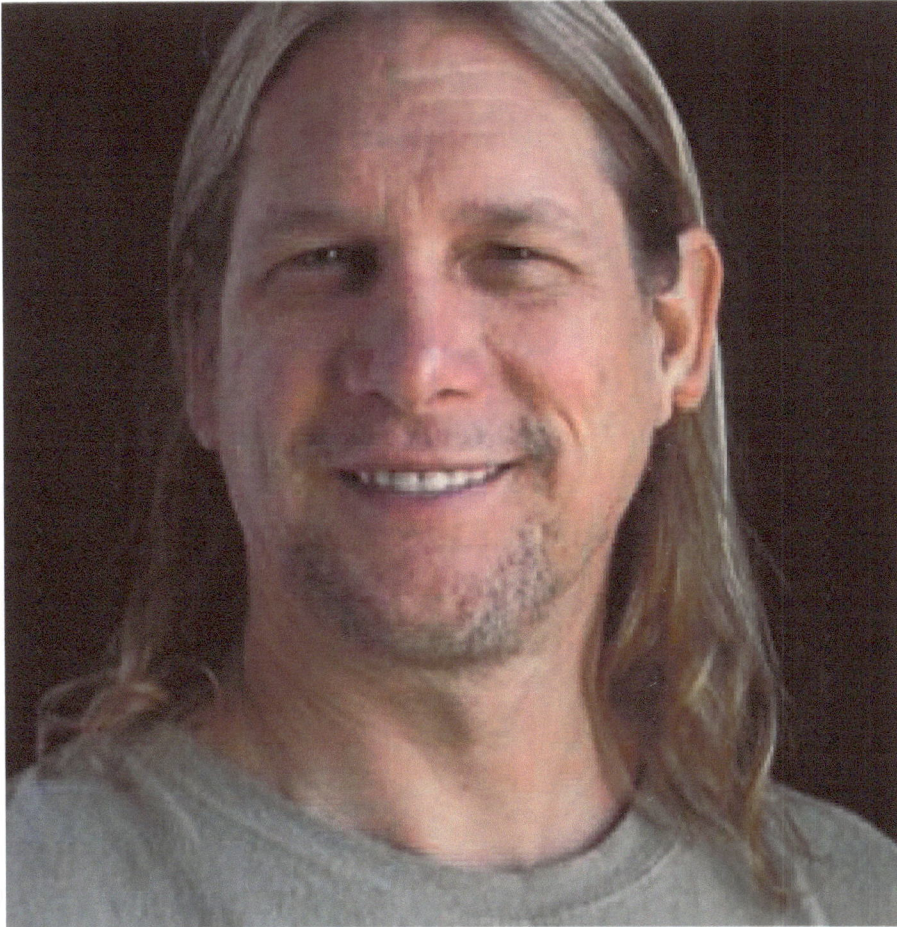

Neha Curtiss
The Director and Teacher
Healing Hands School of Holistic Health,
Escondido, California, USA.

"Thanks to Neha, who passed the Art of Healing
From his hands to mine."
—Nina Bhoot

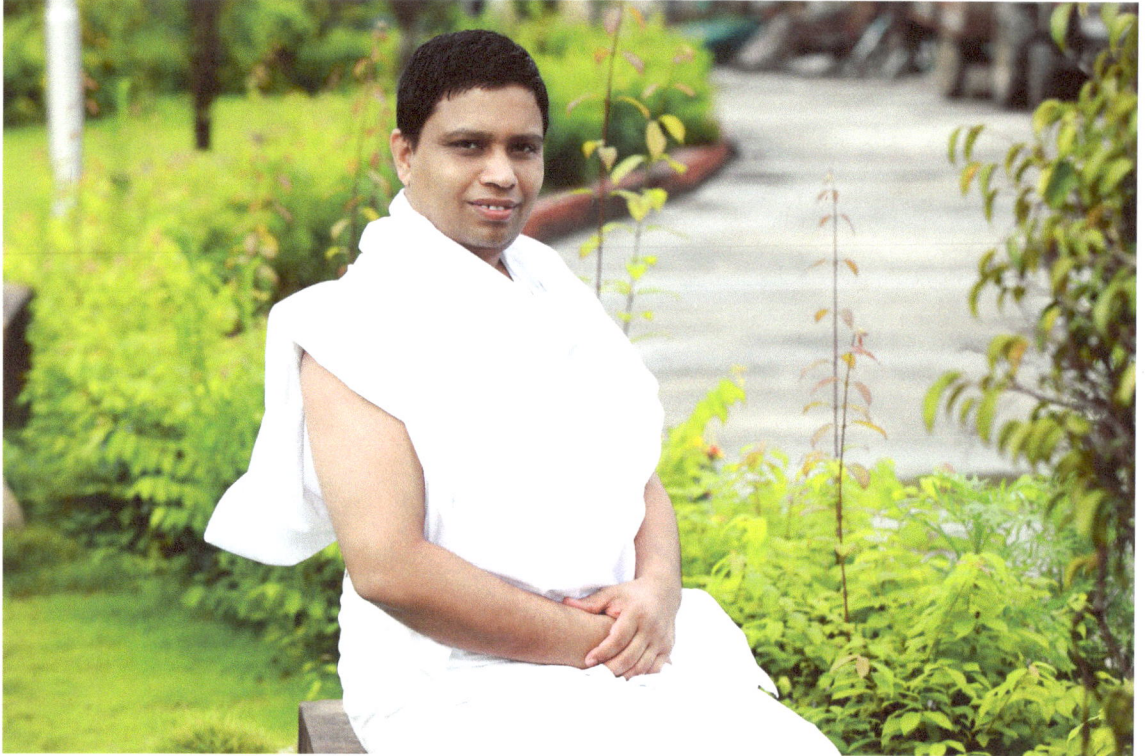

Acharya Sri Balkrishna

The Master of Ayurveda and Secretory General,
Patanjali Yogpeeth, Haridwar, India,
The one who inspired me to put down in writing
My knowledge and experience
In the field of
Structural Body Work /Rolfing.
And this book is the outcome.
I am thankful to him for his support
and encouragement in this work

— Nina Bhoot

FOREWORD

The pains and diseases are more often the result of some kind of inner disorder or imbalance. And there are many kinds therapies invented by mankind to recover from such disorders. Structural Body Work' is one of them. Its concept seems to be similar to the concepts of Yog. I believe this book will be useful for those who are looking forward for better health and so also for yog-students who have difficulties to perform Yog-asanas.

I bless 'Tulsi' Nina for the success of this book.

—**Swami Ramdev** (Yoga Guru)
President, Patanjali Yogpeeth, Haridwar, India

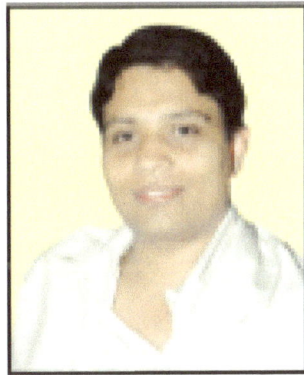

Acharya Sri Balkrishna

'Tulsi' Nina has been working as Holistic Health Practitioner in CA. for many years. She has been known as a 'Healer'. Lately, she has been serving in Patanjali Yogpeeth. A student from Gurukul (of Patanjali Yogpeeth) was suffering from **5 bulging** discs after a serious accident. He was bedridden for a month. None of the Medical or other treatments helped him. Finally, he was sent by an ambulance to 'Tulsi' Nina.

She worked on him continuously for 4 hours; and he was out of bed and walking. There after she worked on him for several weeks and he was totally cured.

This book could be useful for the students of Structural Work as well as patients.

—**Acharya Sri Balkrishna**
Secretary General, Patanjali Yogpeeth, Haridwar, India.

PREFACE

WRITERS REPUBLIC L.L.C.
515 Summit Ave. Unit R1
Union City, NJ 07087, USA

Website: *www.writersrepublic.com*
Hotline: *1-877-656-6838*
Email: *info@writersrepublic.com*

Ordering Information:
Quantity sales. Special discounts are available on quantity purchases by corporations, associations, and others. For details, contact the publisher at the address above.

Printed and bound in the United States of America.

Library of Congress Control Number: 2019947013
ISBN-13:   978-1-64620-011-5   [Paperback Edition]
              978-1-64620-012-2   [Hardback Edition]
              978-1-64620-013-9   [Digital Edition]

Rev. date: 07/22/2019

Synthesis of

STRUCTURAL
BODY WORK

and

YOGA

Based on

ROLFING

Author

Nina Bhoot

Synthesis of **STRUCTURAL BODY WORK**
and **YOGA** based on **ROLFING**

INTRODUCTION

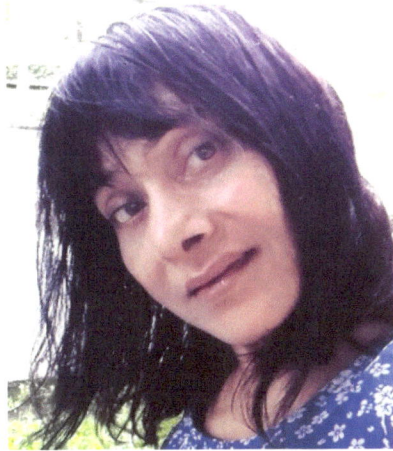

I was gazing the ocean at Laguna Beach that evening. I had left behind me the carriers of Nursing & Med. Asst. and jobs in diverse fields. I always felt, "This is not for me."

Suddenly, Fred, a friend of mine, came back from his long hours of treasure hunting on the beach. He looked miserable. "Oh, my back is hurting" he said. I got up, I put my hand on his back, spontaneously. "I am sorry Fred, that you are in pain" I said. He took a deep breath, and said, "Nina, you have healing hands. Try massage business and you will find job in any corner of the world"

I did not know what he meant, but I took his advice, became LMT and then HHP, in the field of Structural Body Work (Rolfing); and soon, his words became a prophesy. Not only in CA but also in the counties I visited, my hands were appreciated for healing.

This work of manual therapy changed my life. This is like ever learning process, as there is always a possibility to discover more mysteries hidden in Human Body. After more than ten years of my experience in this field, I am still learning. I love my work. Work is my prayer, my Sadhana, the means of personal progress. My work also it changed the life of many people. It is truly said, *'We touch lives, we touch hearts.'*

Synthesis of STRUCTURAL BODY WORK and YOGA based on ROLFING

CONTENTS

PREFACE

PART ONE: BASIC UNDERSTANDING
Basic Understanding of Structural Body Work (SBW)

SBW is a modern Manual Therapy which includes the following:

Science, Occult Science, Concept of Art, Psychosomatic element, Holistic System, the Principle of the Law of Gravity, Consciousness or Awareness (of the therapist and patient/health aspirant) and its Focus is Musculoskeletal Disorders *(MSDs)*

What we understand by Manual Therapy?

A manual therapy is one in which, first, an assessment of the condition of the body is made by observation of posture, gait, movement, range of motion, muscles, soft tissue, and the symptoms. Then on bases of the assessment a treatment is given by using specific manual techniques, in order to release pain, prevent pain or injury, improve physical function, movement, flexibility, protect natural healthy function of the body, help rehabilitation or improve health from good to better.

Structural Body Work (SBW) is a branch of science

What we call Science is a utilitarian knowledge acquired through observation and systematic study and experimentation, and deriving or showing the operation of general laws of any specific subject or matter.

SBW can involve a kind of Occult Science.

Occult science, in brief, is a knowledge and intentional use of invisible powers, forces, energies. For example, Prana Shakti or Chi, intention or will, compassion or love, etc.

Understanding of the concept of Art helps us to do our best:

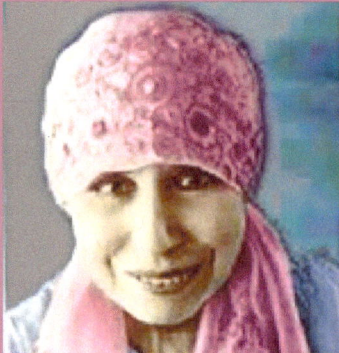

The Mother (1878-1973)
Born in France

Art is not just a skill or talent.

"Art is a living harmony and beauty that must be expressed in all the movements of existence."

—**The Mother** (3.108)
Sri Aurobindo's Ashram, Pondicherry, India

SBW is also a Psychosomatic Therapy:

Any therapy or healing system that includes the following four elements is considered psychosomatic:

1. Consciousness / awareness is the major instrument used in the therapy
2. The therapy proceeds with the knowledge of anatomy, physiology and pathology
3. It insists on the inner experience of the patient / the subject
4. The effects of therapy reflect positively on the body and the psychology

According to the above definition, Hatha Yoga is the most ancient psychosomatic therapy. But there are simile and difference between the concepts and practice of Hatha Yoga and SBW.

Similarities between SBW and Hatha Yoga

For serious Yoga practices, one has to be initiated by a master. But so far as basic physical practices (like Asanas, Shodhan Kriya, (detoxification), Pranayama (regulation of life energy) etc. are concerned, you need to be guided by an expert Yoga Teacher. He may give demo and instructions but does not need to touch your body; and the yoga is supposed to be practiced regularly. It is self-imposed discipline and life style. The goal of yoga is to attain the mastery over body, mind emotions and discover true happiness, love and **freedom**. The practical side effects of yoga are healthy state of body & mind, good posture, and slim body.

Concept of SBW is derived from or influenced by the concept of Yoga. The goal of SBW is to gain better health, to be free from chronic pains or deformation of the body. Positive thoughts & emotions are the side effects of SBW. For the best result in SBW you need a Rolfer or body worker who, with your consent and conscious cooperation, works manually on your body, to help you attain a healthy state. It helps to improve your posture and releases pains. SBW is generally accomplished in 10 sessions within 10 weeks. And the result is often long lasting. *(Please also see p.52)*

Generally, Yoga practice gives you the best health and good posture and keeps you free from pains. However, pain can develop after **whiplash, accident or injury**. SBW can restore a pain-free state.

Structural Body Work is also a Holistic Therapy:

Philosophically, holistic is characterized by the belief that the parts of the being are intimately interconnected and explicable only by reference to the whole.

Medically, holistic is characterized by the treatment of the whole person, considering the psychological and social factors, rather than just the symptoms of a disease.

SBW is Holistic in a sense that it takes into consideration your body with all its part, your psychology (thoughts, emotions and spirit that makes you feel as a whole person).

Any range of medical therapies that are not regarded as 'Allopathic' by the medical profession is considered either Holistic or Alternative

Holistic & Alternative Systems of Medicine/ Therapies

An alternative system of medicine refers to any branch of healing system other than Allopathic. Thus, all the holistic therapies or treatments are considered alternative; alternative to Modern Medicine. *But all Alternative treatments are not holistic*. For example, physical therapy, general massages or other treatments done by machines including General Chiropractic.

According to the above definitions of Holistic, Yoga and Ayurveda are the most ancient holistic systems. Naturopathy as well as all the therapies derived, directly or indirectly, from the concepts of Yoga and Ayurveda are considered to be Holistic. (The source of holistic treatments is given on page p. 65)

Other Holistic Therapies are Homeopathy, Chinese medicine, Acupuncture, Cranio-Sacral, Myofascial Release, modern manual therapies or massage *with an* understanding of exactly *how the touch with different manual techniques affects the body* and mind. (*More understanding about Holistic is given on p. 62*)

As we stated above, certain modern massages are also considered Holistic, we may want to know the difference between massage and SBW.

Difference between Massage and SBW

A massage may give you instant relief but it may not always last long, while SBW gives, often, the lasting solutions for many ailments like chronic pains, spinal or cervical issues etc.

A massage may relieve physical or mental tension, but SBW removes the cause of the tension that is deeper within. A massage could be therapeutic, but it cannot retrain the body how to keep itself balanced. With SBW, the body learns to be balanced and in good poise. Massage does not transform the body, SBW does transforms the body's structure and posture. It helps the body to be aware of its own deeper consciousness. The wrong postures and unhealthy movements, the cause of pain, discomfort and disease disappear after the SBW.

THE PRIMARY FOCUS OF SBW IS

The Mechanical Disorders of Musculoskeletal System (MSDs)

What are Musculoskeletal Disorders (MSDs)?

Musculoskeletal disorders are conditions that can affect your muscles, bones, joints and nerves with a verity of symptoms. The severity of MSDs can vary. In some cases, they cause pain and discomfort that interferes with daily activities.

Symptoms of MSDs can include the following:

Migraine, cervical pain, bulging disk, scoliosis, kyphosis, lordosis, pain in shoulders, wrists, back, hips, legs, knees, feet, short leg syndrome, dull ache, recurrent pain; or pain and discomfort in walking, typing, standing, sitting; or limited srange of motion, shortness of breath, sleep problems (and more, please see 'the misalignment of Atlas' page 44)

It may also involve Neuropathy as follows:

Carpal tunnel syndrome, golfer's elbow, tennis elbow, sciatica, tingling pain, numbness, or weakness in the feet and hands, digestive or cardiovascular problems including blood pressure and other functions, compression of a nerve in the leg, Bell's palsy, the compression of a nerve deforming face, ctc.

The causes of MSDs could be the following:

Lifestyle, activity level, occupation, bad posture at work, sitting in the same position at a computer every day, repetitive motions, lifting heavy weights, a physically idle life, accident, whiplash, emotional trauma, or birth trauma, etc.

MSDs are diagnosed or assessed by examining postural balance, gait, pain, muscle weakness, range of motion, swelling, muscle atrophy, MRI, etc.

HOLISTIC AND ALTERNATIVE TREATMENTS FOR MSDs
(depending on severity of the case)

1. **Physical therapy,** Myofascial Release, Moderate exercise, Yoga, Improving lifestyle

2. **Deep Tissue** or other Massages, as may be necessary for occasional pains

3. **Chiropractic:** in case of acute pain, or pains from heavy exercise, sports or the cases of moderate to severe problems.

4. **Structural Body Work or Rolfing:** in case of whiplash, slipped/bulging disc, spinal deformations, chronic pains, recurring pains, or when no other treatment gives a lasting improvement.

THE FOCUS OF CHIROPRACTIC IS ALSO MSDs

But there is some similarity and difference between the two, as follows:

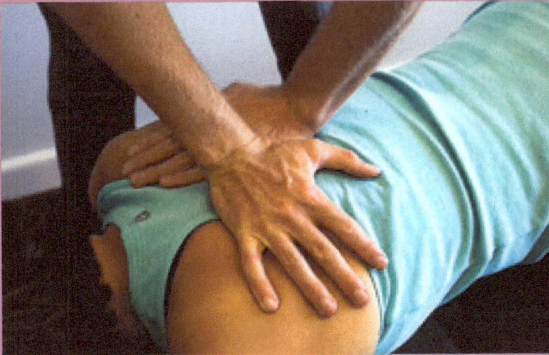

Similarities, Chiropractic & SBW

Both are manual therapies that help to relieve pains from MSDs. They are better alternatives to pain killers; have no side effects and they help to stop or slow down the degenerative disease.

Difference, Chiropractic and SBW

Chiropractic is considered alternative medicine while SBW is Holistic. Approaches of Chiropractic and Structural Body Work are different and so also their outcome. The Chiropractor adjusts the spine or brings the vertebra or joints into alignment directly by pressing or pushing them in appropriate direction. It gives you instant relief. But if the cause of misalignment is muscular/ fascial tension, the bones go out of alignment periodically. So, you may need to go to Chiropractor more often. SBW on the other hand, works on spine indirectly, works on the whole body-fascia slowly over a period of time, to release the tension in the whole fascial network which is the cause of misalignment. As a result, the patient/health aspirant has better posture with the benefits of lasting solution for pain.

WHEN TO GO FOR CHIROPRACTIC?

Chiropractic is excellent for acute pain or sudden discomfort form certain movement, exercise, sport or other activity. It can give you immediate cure or relief.

In case of chronic pain or discomfort, go to chiro after getting "deep tissue" or other medical massage therapies that would release muscular tension first, so that the chiropractic adjustment would last longer. You can have better result if a 'good experienced' masseuse and chiropractor coordinate with each other.

SBW would be excellent when there is no cure or lasting relief by Chiro-specifically in chronic or recurrent pains, whiplash consequences, disc problems, or other MSDs not much improved by other systems of medicine, or ***Allopathy***

ALLOPATHY

It is worthwhile for the Structural Body Workers or those working in different holistic or alternative field, and so also for the patients /health aspirants, having basic understanding about specialty of Allopathic Medicine as well as its limitations.

Specialty of Allopathy:

Medical Diagnosis *is an excellent help.*

Medical diagnosis can be useful also to 'health care providers' and therapists working in Alternative or Holistic Health field. For example, it may help Structural Body Worker to know when he should not take the case, or specific precautions he may have to take during the treatment. Massage therapist may find it helpful to learn the type of massage or pressure required in a given condition; a naturopath may know from medical diagnosis that certain diseases may not have a solution even in naturopathy, a physical therapist may learn better the pros and cons of the therapy in a given condition. **Therefore,** it is good idea to have a glance on patient/health aspirant's Medical History before starting any treatment.

In Emergency, Allopathic medicine can save your life

It stops spreading contagious diseases and epidemics

Surgery is excellent if it is used when absolutely necessary

Limitations of Allopathic Medicine

- There is no cure for most diseases;
- Allopathic approach seeks to manage disease lifelong.
- Negative side effects of the allopathic drugs may cause many secondary problems.

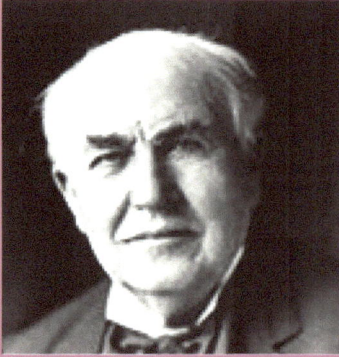

Thomas Edison

"The doctor of the future will not prescribe drugs. Instead, he will awaken the interest of the patient towards his body, as well as to the reason and the possibility of preventing the disease."

—Thomas Edison
Inventor and Businessman, USA

DR. IDA ROLF

The inventor of "Rolfing" or Structural Integration (SBW)

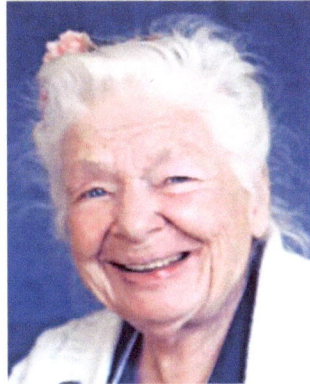

Dr. Ida Rolf (1896- 1979)

In the East, specifically in India, the science of physical and mental health and healing was known in the form of Yoga and Ayurveda since time immemorial. After the Islamic invasion and later by British colonization the Vedic science and Art were buried. The culture of Yoga and Ayurveda was revived by the struggle of Hatha Yoga Guru Swami Ramdev and Acharya Balakrishna (supported by many Hindu organizations.)

In the West, specifically in USA, the people had been looking towards the East to find alternative therapies, like massage, Yoga, Ayurveda, or healing in natural ways. A few of those, inspired from Yoga, invented new alternative healing systems. One of them was Dr. Ida Rolf.

According to the article "Yoga and prevention of injury", the concept of Yoga was the major factor in Dr. Ida's early understanding of human body and mind. Yoga was Dr. Ida's organizing principle, in her career as therapist.

Dr. Ida Rolf believed that Yoga was the best physical culture ever known by humanity.

She had been studying Yoga for years. She was the student of 'Pier B.' who was a Tantric Yogi. The principle of 'Vertical Axis' in Structural Integration is believed to be inspired from him. Keeping in mind the traditional goal of Yoga, the goal of structural integration was defined, and **she invented an original technique or working process for Structural Integration.**

'Fascia' is the discovery of Dr. Ida Rolf, and it is a great contribution towards science of anatomy and physiology and pathology. The organizing of fascia is also the focal point in Structural Integration (or SBW). Later, inspired by the principle of organizing fascia, many other therapies were invented, e.g. Mayo Fascial Release, The Feldenkrais Method, Alexander Technique, Palates, Structural Yoga Etc.

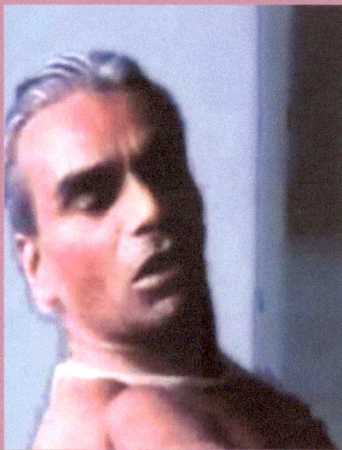

Yogi Iyengar, (1918 - 2014)

Yogi BSK Iyengar is known to be one of the pioneers who brought Yoga to the West. When he was born, Ida Rolf was 22 years old. Thus, she was an advocate of Yoga practices before Yogi Iyengar came into picture.

"Yoga allows you to discover a sense of wholeness in your life, where you do not feel like you are constantly trying to fit broken pieces together."

—Yogi BSK Iyengar

You could feel a sense of wholeness after Rolfing or Structural Body Work, too.

PRE-REQUIREMENTS
For the Students of Structural Body Work

1. **Knowledge of**:

   Anatomy, the science of the shape and structure of the body and its parts

   Physiology, the science of the function and movements of the body and its parts

   Pathology, the branch of science that studies the nature of disease, its causes, and development, the nature of diseases that are caused by structural imbalance or musculoskeletal disorders, nature of functional changes caused by structural changes, structural and functional changes created by particular disease.

2. **Deep Tissue Manipulation (DTM)**: Must have taken the course of DTM prior to SBW. Some therapists have the misconception that the Deep Tissue is a kind of massage with hard pressure. You must have a clear understanding of the concept the Deep Tissue and its technique and experience, without which you may cause injury.

3. **Structural Analysis:** The classes 'Structural Analysis' are very useful in this work. These classes are about learning the geometry of the body in relation to three planes, and be able to spot the misalignments, or deformations, and to visualize the aligned structure.

4. **Massage Experience:** Knowledge and experience of massage, in general, is **helpful**, since the hands already "know" the art of touch.

5. **The knowledge of good Customer Service** and the **skill of nonviolent communication** is very helpful. It makes the client receptive, and the receptivity is of vital importance in SBW.

6. **Understanding "Emotional Release",** since nine out of ten clients have emotional release during the course of SBW.

WHAT IS EMOTIONAL RELEASE? *

According to the modern discovery made by Dr. Upledger, the memories of the experience of life, forgotten from the conscious mind, are stored or "saved' in the cells of the body. In yogic language the memories are registered in the vital or subconscious level of the being. It is called 'Samskara' in Sanskrit language.

When these stored memories are of a serious accident or mental or emotional trauma, they have negative influence on our personality. They influence our behavior, thinking and emotions but we are not conscious of it. When we go through SBW or any psychosomatic therapy, the dormant memories are suddenly awakened.

In other words, when the part of your body where the memories were stored, is contacted by the therapist, the client suddenly remembers the past experience. At that moment either tears roll down from his eyes or he bursts into crying, or he may want to narrate the story of the past trauma. This experience is called "Emotional Release".

Emotional Release is a very important event in the process of SBW because the negative memories that affected the person's behavior or physical health are released in this way, thereby the person is free form the negative behavior or ill-health.

* Craniosacral therapists call it as "Somato Emotional Release" or SRE as coined by Dr. Upledger.

DUTIES OF THE THERAPIST
WHEN THE CLIENT IS HAVING AN EMOTIONAL RELEASE

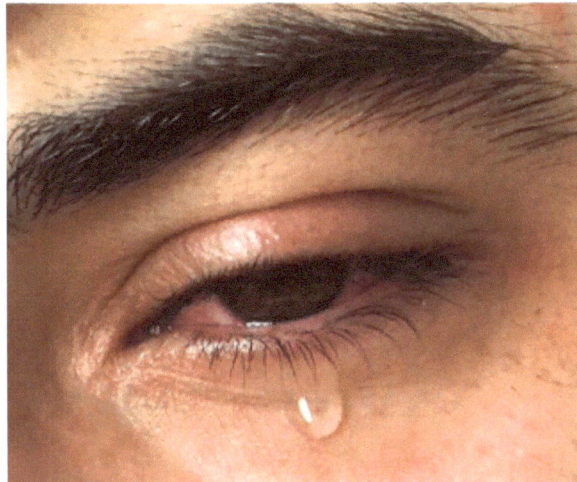

- Remain calm, never be surprised.
- Do not ask the client, "Are OK?" or "What happened?"
- Let him cry as much as he feels like and tell him that crying is good for him.
- Be compassionate and kind.
- Listen to the client attentively; don't be judgmental; do not comment.
- Keep the contact of your hand on his/her body
- When he/she becomes calm, continue the treatment.

INTERESTING STORIES OF DORMANT MEMORIES:

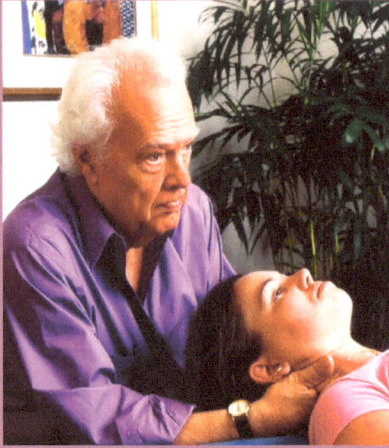
Dr. Upledger

A lady was always suffering from suicidal thoughts. She decided to get Craniosacral therapy (an invention of Dr. Upledger)

During the session she went into deep sleep and she remembered hearing the voice of her grandmother while she was in her mother's womb. Grandma was scolding her mom and wanted her go for abortion.

This lady understood the cause of her suicidal thoughts. She forgave her Granma and was free from ideas of suicide.

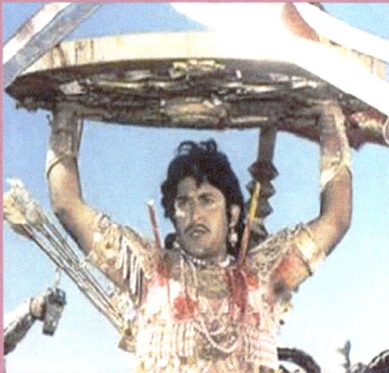
Abhimanyu

This reminds us the story of Abhimanyu, one of the great heroes of Mahabharata, the first world war, (technically, 16 Oct. to 3 Nov. 5561 B.C).

It is recorded that he happened to 'remember' later in his life the war- strategy of 'Chakra-Vyuha' which he heard while he was in his mother Subhadra's womb when Arjuna, his father was explaining the strategy.

The modern discovery of Dr. Upledger is an affirmation of truth in the ancient stories (There are many such stories)

These stories may give a hint to pregnant women that they can positively influence the character of the child in womb, if they want.

STORED MEMORIES
The Statements of Genius People

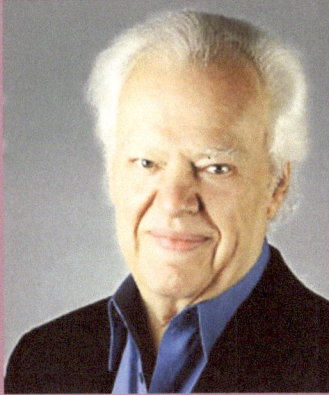

*"The memories are
stored in the cells of the body."*

—Dr. Upledger

*Sri Aurobindo had stated the same fact, in different
words, long before Dr. Upledger.*

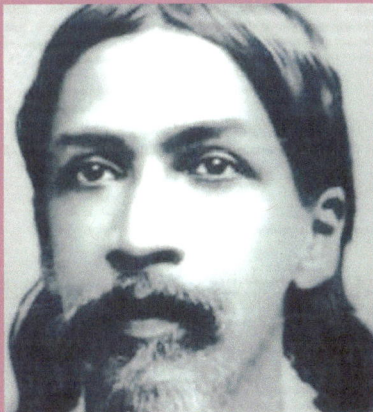

Dr. (Surgeon) Upledger (USA)

*"Memory is everywhere,
even if you are conscious of it or not...
but everything (you experienced)
is stored in Prana,
the basic stuff of consciousness...*

even the feet have the memories of their own."

—Sri Aurobindo

Sri Aurobindo

According to the Mother,
The memories of all lives on earth are registered in the matter of earth.

(Question and answer 1953)

PART TWO: THE THEORY

The Theory of Structural Body Work

The Theory of Structural Body Work is based on five principles as following:

1. The force of Gravity
2. Geometry of the Body
3. Fascia and Skeleton
4. Movement
5. Touch and Consciousness or Awareness

1st Principle of SBW:
THE FORCE OF GRAVITY

"The most essential characteristics of all biological systems are defined by the Universal Law of Gravity."
— (by an author unknown)

The Gravity of earth is an inevitable force that affects our existence at every moment of our life. It influences our body and mind constantly, but we are hardly aware of it. The Force of Gravity is a physical fact and a spiritual reality; or we may say they are two sides of a coin. The ignorance of the 'effect of the gravity' on us, is major cause of our most of the pains. The Yoga-Sutra of ancient Yogi Patanjali states, *"Avidya Kshetram Uttaresham"* *"Ignorance is the cause of the rest of the causes of pain"* may also apply here, as the rest of the four principles of SBW are related to the Gravity.

What is the Gravity?

- Gravity in general, is a force of attraction between any two objects with mass *(from smallest atoms to the greatest objects in the galaxies)* It is a natural phenomenon. Here we are concerned with the gravity of earth.
- Gravity is the cause of Evolution on earth, from matter to life to mind.
- Dr. Ida Rolf believed that there is something in the universe that attracts the beings on earth to rise against the gravity, yet she could not define it. *(But it is defined in old Indian Literature)*

THE RELATIONSHIP:
Animal Body & Human Body with the Earth & Gravity

The spine of the animals is more or less horizontal to the surface of earth. An animal-body finds in its own way, its harmony with the force of gravity. The structure of animal-body and its movement in space is in coordination with the force of gravity. It moves with ease, e.g. flying of bird in sky, gliding of fish in water, movement snake, jumping of monkeys, dancing of peacock, running of wild animal, etc., is so gracious, beautiful and divine. How about human?

The spine of the human is made to stay vertical. This is very important Event in the course of Evolution on earth (materially and spiritually) The spine being vertical and the body having a high center of gravity on a very small base, with the head on the top to be balanced between the shoulders, it is less easy to keep the body in harmony with the force of gravity.

Maybe mankind needs to evolve further to discover better balance or it is an indication that the human evolution is not yet complete!

CONCEPTS OF EVOLUTION: EAST & WEST
Modern Theory of Evolution, Myth or Truth?

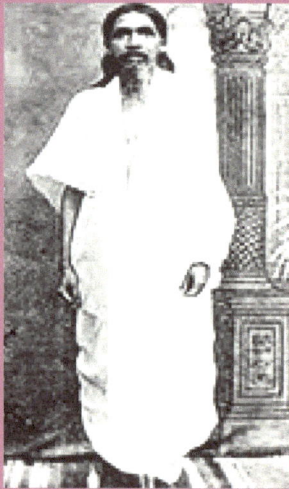

Manu to Man

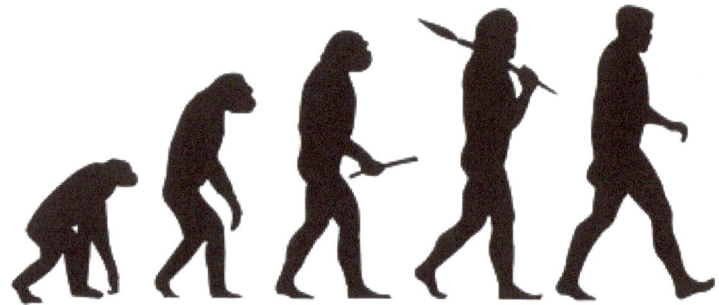

Monkey to man, the Hypothesis (a myth)

According to modern **hypothesis**, the ancestor of man is **'believed'** to be monkey, though there is no evidence, which they call the **"Missing Link"** found yet. "And they will never find it" said the Mother, "as the first man was precipitated in the Subtle Physical."

It is mentioned in the Vedic literature that 'the ancestor of Man was Manu'. The Sanskrit word "Manav" (Man) literary means "The descendent of Manu, a mental being."

20

CONCEPT OF EVOLUTION IN VEDA
(The most ancient Hindu Scripture)

What the modern science discovered recently about the evolution had been already stated in Vedic literature. The Puranic stories of Dashavatar, (fish, amphibian, animal, half-animal half-man, undeveloped man, and progressively more evolved men) is symbol of evolution from less evolved life to more developed beings. And the story does not end there. It also indicates (in Rigveda) the future, a Supramental evolution of mankind. *(Refer Sri Aurobindo's literature)*

The continuity of the evolution of Mankind

Most of the animal babies start walking very soon after they are born. Below we examine the stages between the sitting, standing and walking of a child. There is slow and steady changes or transformation also in structure and posture. It takes a long time (comparatively) before a child can walk properly.

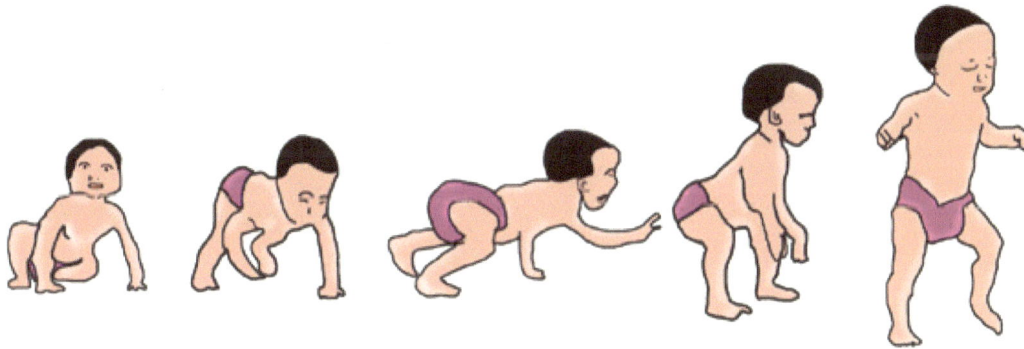

According to yogic concept, the transformation in the structure of the body follows, in reality, the transformation of the consciousness of the being.

An animal is perfect in itself and it has attained its perfection, thus, the animal has stopped its evolution. Human being is not perfect (unfortunately or fortunately) and to attain his own perfection he has to raise himself to a higher Consciousness first, and ultimately to evolve towards Superman. *(Reference: Sri Aurobindo's literature)*

SBW, Structural Changes & Change in Consciousness

According to the Vedic literature, *Energy (Shakti) is the source of Matter.* (In other words, the Matter is the condensed form of Energy. Modern science has discovered recently the same.) *And the source of energy is 'Chitta' the 'Consciousness',* (which the modern science has not yet discovered)

In brief:

Consciousness transforms into → **Energy** transfers into → **Matter**

If the above statement is true, then reverse is also possible as follows:

Matter (in the material body) → (could awaken the internal) **Energy** by touch →
→ to awake **the Consciousness of the body** (to change the) → **Matter** (material body)

The process of 'Structural Body Work' seems to follow the path as stated above.

CENTER OF GRAVITY, LINE OF GRAVITY & ITS PLACE IN HUMAN BODY

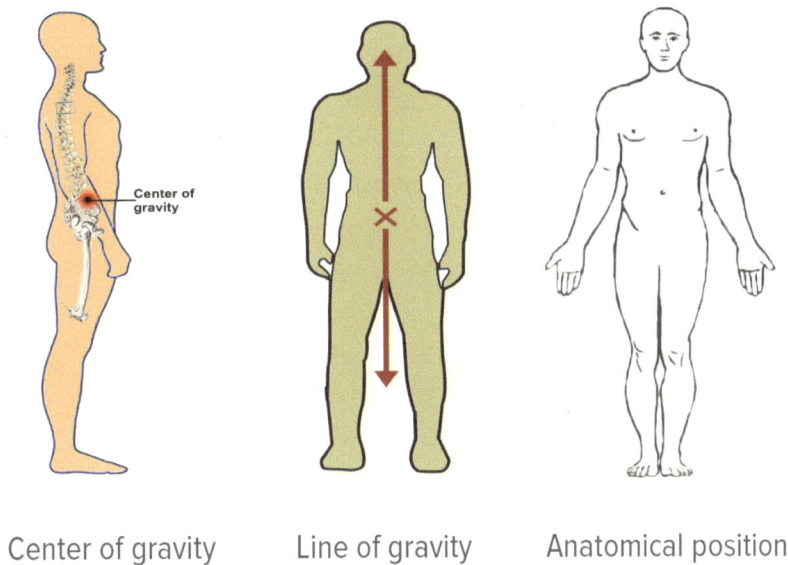

Center of gravity   Line of gravity   Anatomical position

- ***The Center of Gravity*** is a point in the body, around which the mass or weight of the body is evenly distributed, and through which the force of gravity acts.

- It is the point where the weight of the body is centered and all the parts of the body are considered balanced around it.

- The center of gravity is the point where the sum of the distributed mass of the body is zero.

- The center of gravity in human body is located in front of the second sacral vertebrae when the body is in the anatomical position.

- So long as the structure of the body is balanced; the center of gravity does not shift.

- When the body is in motion, the center of gravity may be outside of the body, and it depends on the relation of the different parts of the body with each other.

- The center of gravity shifts by changing the position of arms and legs.
- Carrying weight shifts the center of gravity
- Amputation of any part of the body shifts the body's center of gravity.
- The effect of the gravity in relation to any part of the body is measured in relation to the vertical line of gravity

The Line of Gravity, in the anatomical position, is an imaginary vertical line which passes from the center of gravity of the body to the center of earth.

Posture is a term used to describe a position of the body or the arrangements of body parts relative to one another and in relation to the vertical Line of Gravity.

WHAT WE MEAN BY 'GOOD POSTURE' IN SBW?

When all the body-parts /blocks are parallel to the Line of Gravity, the body is said to be in good posture. It is ideal. In the state of good posture, the line of Gravity passes through the center of pelvic floor; and the ears, shoulder joints, greater trochanters, knee joints, and ankle joints are located in coronal plane, and the line of gravity looks as the bow of the arc of the spine, in anatomical position.

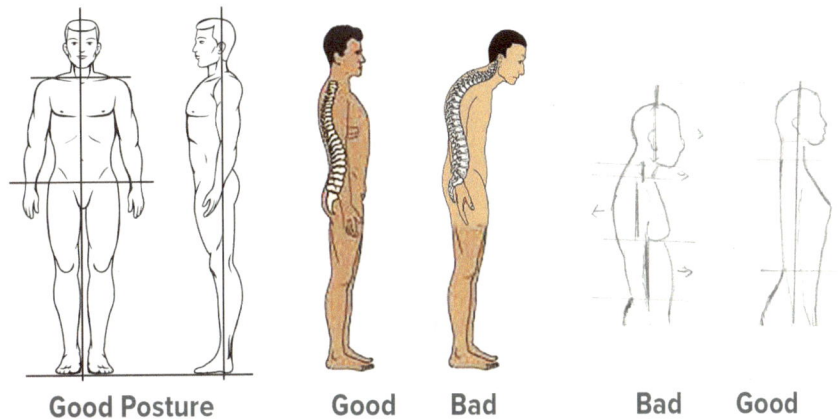

Good Posture   **Good   Bad**   **Bad   Good**

In a state of good posture, the body segments are balanced in the position of least strain and maximum support; there is balance between Muscular System and Skeletal System, and the muscles function most efficiently. So, it conserves energy, protects the body against injury and progressive deformities or degeneration.

Factors affecting posture:

1. **Primary** and **Mechanical** factors: **The relationship of the line of Gravity to body segments**

2. **Anatomical factors**: Integration of Musculoskeletal system

3. **Neural control**, integrity of Musculoskeletal and nervous system

4. **Dental health:** Integrity of teeth, jaw and bite, Temporomandibular joint dysfunction TMJD

5. **Flexibility** of the structure of weight bearing segments

6. **Strength** of antigravity muscles and balance of antagonist muscles

7. **Psychological factors**, such as depression or other emotions or the state of mind.

8. **Visual** and kinesthetic awareness *(Yoga plays role in all of above)*

Dental Health: Alignment of Teeth, Jaw and Posture

Posture and integrity of jaw, teeth and bite are closely related. One affects the other, involving muscles in the neck, back, pelvis and legs. Our bodies have a high center of gravity on a very small base; and the spine is made to be vertical, with head on the top, it requires to be in agreement with the line of gravity; a complicated process!

When your teeth or any part of your body is out of alignment with the other parts, there is a chain reaction; the chain from feet to head, or rather **teeth** (more accurately).

When your upper and lower teeth are closed together, each tooth naturally forms a skeletal relationship with the opposite tooth, and the bite determines the position of your jaw, and in turn, the position of your head on the spine.

Your teeth are part of the skeletal system. When your teeth are misaligned, there is compressive effect, or chain reaction throughout the posture. So the body will try to adjust itself, involving muscles of the neck, back, pelvis, leg and feet, resulting bad posture or postural deformations.

TMJD involves various components of the masticatory system, muscles, nerves, tendons, ligaments, bones, connective tissue. The cause of TMJD is often considered idiopathic. But it is often believed to be related to musculoskeletal, psychosomatic and autoimmune disorders.

How do we use SBW to attain a Good Posture and get relief from pains or MSDs?

- By bringing balance and integrity between Muscular and Skeletal system
- Align the body segments parallel to the Line of Gravity
- Improving flexibility, strength and neuromuscular coordination
- Consequently, it helps to uplift the emotions and changes the psychological state.

WHAT ARE THE BENEFITS OF SBW?

- By SBW, most postural problems as well as health can be improved at any age. (However, longer the problem exists, the more difficult it is to correct.)
- Relief from chronic pains.
- Helps to relieve the psychosomatic disorders and promotes a positive attitude
- Improves Flexibility and neuromuscular coordination
- Body conserves energy and feels strong, light and youthful
- Protects the body against injury and progressive deformities or degeneration
- SBW can

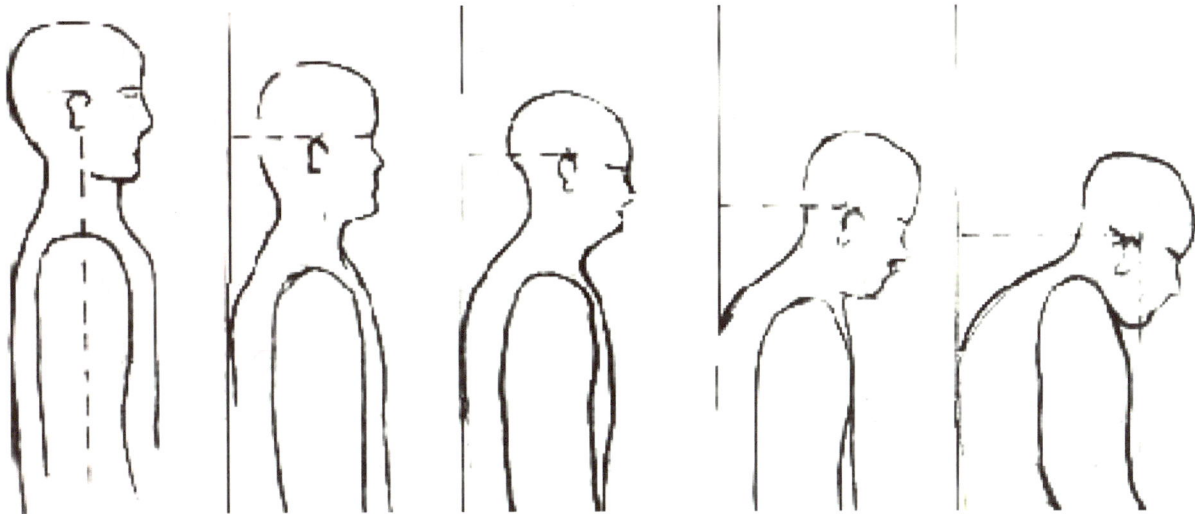

Prevent the Deterioration of Posture

BAD POSTURE AND MSDs

The possibility of ideal posture or a balance state of the body is given to us by Natural Evolution. The body from childhood to adulthood is generally, very flexible balanced and full of energy. It moves in space with ease. If the conscious care of the body, its posture and movement is taken, (by Yoga, exercise, or other physical discipline and awareness), the flexibility and energy level could be maintained for a long time.

Unfortunately, most people begin to lose their natural balance around the age of forty or fifty. Some people, who have been able to maintain the balance by efforts, also lose it at some point of life, and become hard, imbalanced and disorganized. Tension or injury or deformation in any part of the body results in chain reaction throughout the body causing deformation of the posture, or Musculoskeletal Disorder (MSD). The harmony between the different parts of the body is compromised; the movement is no longer effortless. The center of gravity of the body is shifted in proportion to the postural deformation. Fatigue of the body in movement is in proportion to the shift of the center of gravity, because the body is in constant war with the force of gravity and to fight with the gravity of earth is a sure way to be defeated.

The causes of MDSs, illness, tension and deformation of posture:

Physical causes: Life style, habit of wrong postures at work, absence of physical discipline, excessive physical efforts, wrong way of exercising or gym activity, whiplash or accident, lack of necessary rest, serious illness, too many allopathic drugs, unnecessary surgeries, malnutrition, junk food etc.

Obesity leads to enhance the normal vertebral column curves, resulting in the development of abnormal or excessive curvatures. The accumulation of body weight in the abdominal region results an anterior shift in the Line of Gravity that carries the weight of the body. This causes in an anterior tilt of the pelvis and a pronounced enhancement of the lumbar curve like lordosis, or swayback.

Psychological causes: Mental stress, emotional trauma, fear etc.

Subconscious causes: Collective suggestions

RELATED QUOTES

Allopathic Medicine & Doctors

"I have no preference for allopathic... the doctors very usually make thing worse instead for better by spoiling nature's resistance to illness by excessive and ill-directed use of medicines..."

* * *

— **Sri Aurobindo**

Fear

"In fact, 90% of illnesses are the result of the subconscious fear of the body.

In ordinary consciousness, the fear is more or less a hidden anxiety about the consequences of the slightest physical disturbance. It can be translated by these words of doubt about the future. "And what will happen?" It is this anxiety that must be checked. Indeed, this anxiety is a lack of confidence in the Divine Grace..."

— **The Mother (15, 151)**

Collective Suggestions

"There are cases of swine flu; it is horrible..." This is a collective suggestion of fear. If your mind or emotion gets into this, you are sure to get the flu. It is true with any disease. Thus, spread the epidemics.

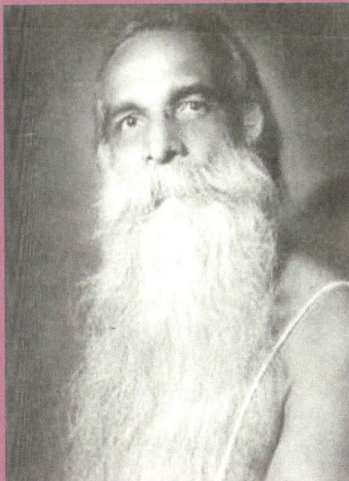

Champaklal

*"Mother, I am fifty,
I think I am getting old"*

— *Champaklal*

*"No, no, my child.
This is a collective suggestion.
Never accept it.*

— *The Mother*
(Sri Aurobindo's Ashram, Pondicherry, India)

IN MSDs OR BAD POSTURE

What is Wrong Anatomically or Physiologically?
And what is the process to correct it?

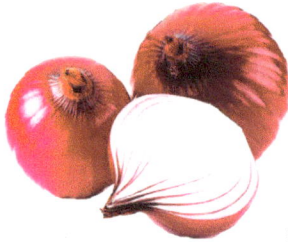

For this purpose, we need first to understand the layers of the muscles. The muscles in the body are arranged in layers (like the layers in the bulb of an onion) and there are subtle layers of fascia between them, separating the layers from each other.

There is also a liquid substance, like gelatin, called ground substance, between the layers of muscles, which helps the muscles to glide over each other during the movement. If a muscle or fascia is pulled or tense, get adhesion or hardened or shortened, the liquid substance between the muscles becomes dry for some reason, then the muscles have difficulty to move or glide over each other. They produce resistance and pain in movement. When the muscles become hard or what we call 'knotted', nerves in the muscles get compressed causing pain. Muscles are attached to the bones, and when muscles are shortened, they pull the bones out of place and deform the structure, cause pressure on nerves and pain.

Superficial Layer and Deeper Layer of Muscles

1. The **layer** of the muscles that support the spine and the core is called Deeper layer of muscles. The layer of muscles that helps to move the body in space is called Superficial layer of muscles.

2. Thus, in general, the muscles of the torso are considered the muscles of deeper layer. The muscles involved in movements of arms and legs (extremities) are considered superficial muscles.

3. Some muscles of the deeper layer help to move the extremities and therefore are considered Superficial; e.g. SCM, Pectoralis, Trapezius and the muscles of arm pit. Some muscles of the superficial layer are

supporting and stabilizing the core, therefore considered Deeper muscles. e.g., Adductors and Subscapularis.

4. The deeper layer is the support of life, and related to "Being"
   The superficial layer is related to "Doing"

5. The characteristic *sense of self* depends on the balance among the muscles of deeper layer, like Psoas, Rectus abs and Diaphragm.

6. The important muscles of the deeper layer are: Psoas, Rectus abs, Diaphragm, iliacus, Rib-muscles, Rotators of Hips, QL, Erector Spinae, Adductors.

7. The important muscles of the superficial layers are: SCM, Pacts, Traps, Latissimus, other thigh muscles.

MORE UNDERSTANDING OF THE SUPERFICIAL AND DEEPER LAYERS OF THE MUSCLES:

Imagine you are walking and suddenly you tripped over something. Your body, without your conscious thought, moves in space to get back into balance, or to protect itself. This movement is initiated by the deeper layer of the muscles. The superficial layer of the muscles works in harmony with the Deeper layer.

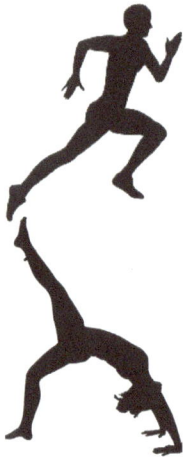

Imagine you are running. The superficial layer of the muscles makes the effort first. You feel some fatigue, and then after some time, the running becomes effortless and pleasant. This is possible when the superficial layer becomes flexible and gives room to the deeper layer to expand. Then the process of running becomes effortless.

The superficial layer of muscles makes the effort first, in the process of Yog-asana. It slowly helps the superficial muscles to be flexible, which gives room to the deeper layer of the muscles and then the 'Asana' becomes effort-less, or "Prayatna-Shaithilyen", as it is stated in Yoga sutra by Maharshi Patanjali.

Co-relation between the Deeper and superficial layers of the muscles

If you put thick and tight gloves on, and try to move your fingers, you will feel resistance, and it is the difficult to do a job with fingers. The superficial muscles are like gloves, when they are tight and hardened, they are resistant. It is difficult for the deeper layers of muscles to function properly. So, you feel discomfort or pain. (or MSD)

To correct MSD, Structural Body Work proceeds in the steps as follows:

1. Release the tension, resistance, adhesion, knots, hardness in the Superficial layer of muscles, (sessions 1, 2, 3)
2. Release tension, contractions, hardness etc. in the deeper layer of muscles (sessions 4, 5, 6, 7)
3. Then integrate superficial layer and the deeper layer of muscles (sessions 8, 9)
4. Total Integration (session 10)

CONCEPTS OF GRAVITY:
ANCIENT YOGIC AND MODERN SCIENTIFIC

(This subject is directly related to Yoga and indirectly to SBW)

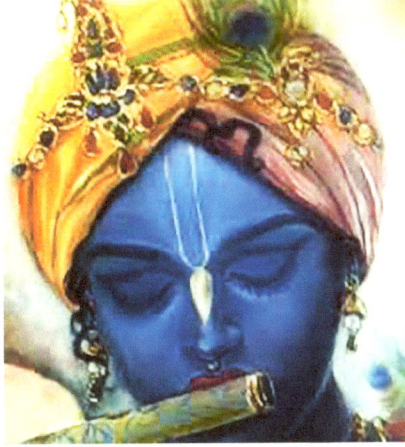

*Thanks to Iskcon for this painting
and Swami Prabhupad who spread the scientific
and spiritual concept of Krishna around the world*

"Sarvam Krishna-mayam jagat" **(Bhagavat Puran)**

"The whole universe is pervaded by "Krishna." The word Krishna is derived from Sanskrit root 'krish' (कृ ष) means to pull, to attract. Thus, t h e meaning o f 'Krishna' is 'All Attractive, the Force of Attraction. So, *"Sarvam krishna-mayam jagat" s* means the whole universe, from an atom to the planets and galaxies, is pervaded by the Force of Attraction, which is The Divine Power of the Supreme Personality, called Krishna, spiritually; and the Force of Gravity, materially.

"Sarava-Bhoota-Sthitam mam..." **(Bhagavat Gita 3/11)**

Krishna, the force of attraction (or gravity) is present in everything.

"Mayi savamidam proktam sutre manigana iva" **(Bhagavat Gita 7/7)**

The whole universe is sustained by Krishan or the Force of Gravity, in the same way as the beads are sustained together by a thread.

"Bijam mam sarva bhootanam viddhi..." **(B. Gita 7/10)**

Know Krishna, or the Force of Gravity as the seed of Creation (and evolution).

FORMULAE FOR DEFYING THE LAW OF GRAVITY

"Kaya-akashayoh-sambandha-samyamat lagutul-samapteh-akash-gamanam."
— (Yoga Sutra of Ancient Yogi Patanjali)

"By doing "Samyama" on the relation between the body and sky (space, ether), the body becomes light and one can fly in the sky."

It is recorded in the history of Rama, that Hanuman flew from India to Sri Lanka, Sri Lanka to Himalaya and back to Sri Lanka. He knew how to play with laws of Gravity, he could make his body light like a feather, or heavy like a mountain (he gave a demo in the court of Ravana, the king of Sri Lanka)

In 13th Century, Sant Yogi Gyaneshwar too, was known to have such power.

LEVITATION
(Defying the law of gravity)

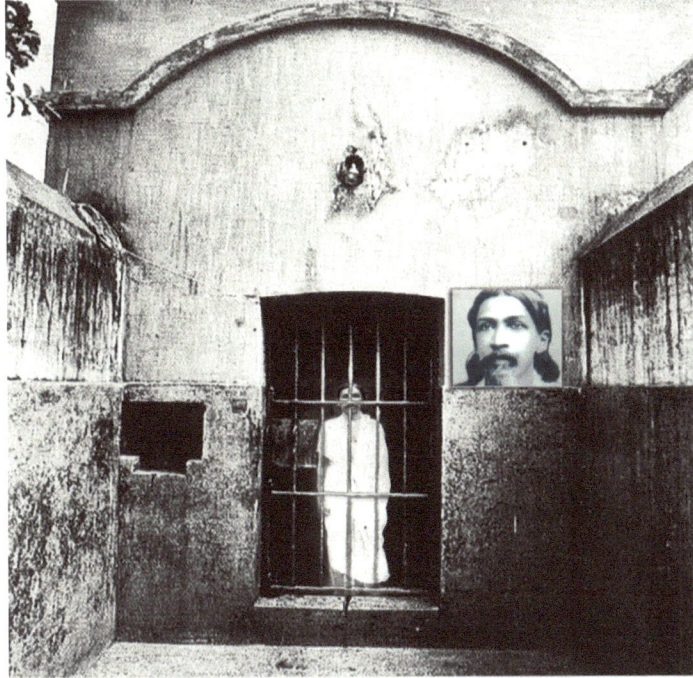

Alipore jail where Sri Aurobindo,
The Great Yogi and Pioneer of Revolutionary Movement to free India
from British Rule, was confined for one year.

"That once happened in Alipore jail (1908-09) I was having very intense Sadhana (Yogic endeavor) on vital plane and I was concentrated, I had questioning mood, whether such Siddhi (power) as Uthapana, (levitation) were possible.

Then suddenly I found myself raised in such a way I could not have done it myself with muscular exertion: Only one part of the body was slightly in contact with the ground and the rest was raised up against the wall and I know I could not have held my body like that normally even if I wanted it."

I found that the body remained suspended like that without any exertion on my part"

— **Sri Aurobindo**

35

2nd Principle of SBW
GEOMETRY OF THE BODY
IN RELATION TO THE GRAVITY

The Concept of Directional Reference:

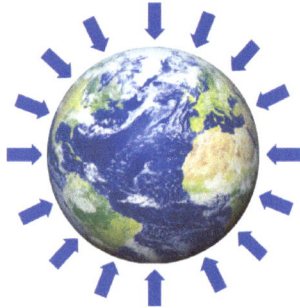

The force of gravity holds us to the surface of earth, and its force works vertically down towards the center of earth. Thus, it gives us the concept of "Down" towards earth and "Up" away from earth.

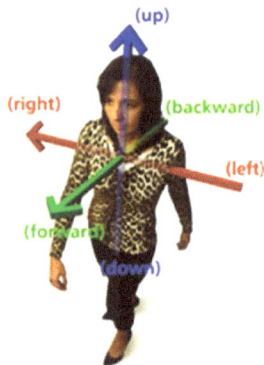

The concept of 'up and down' leads us to the concepts of right and left, as well as front and back. Thus, it gives us the concept of three directional reference; and so also the concept of three planes.

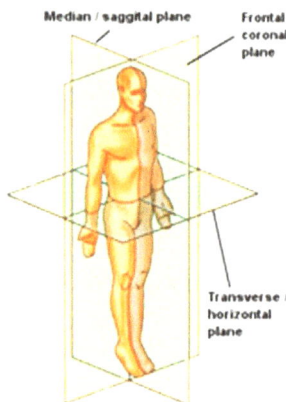

Understanding the three planes of the body

1. **Sagittal Plane** is an imaginary plane that divides the body into right and left halves
2. **Coronal Plane** is an imaginary plane that divides the body into front and back
3. **Transverse Plane** is an imaginary plane that divides the body into upper and lower parts

GOOD POSTURE
In the Relation to the Three Planes of the Body

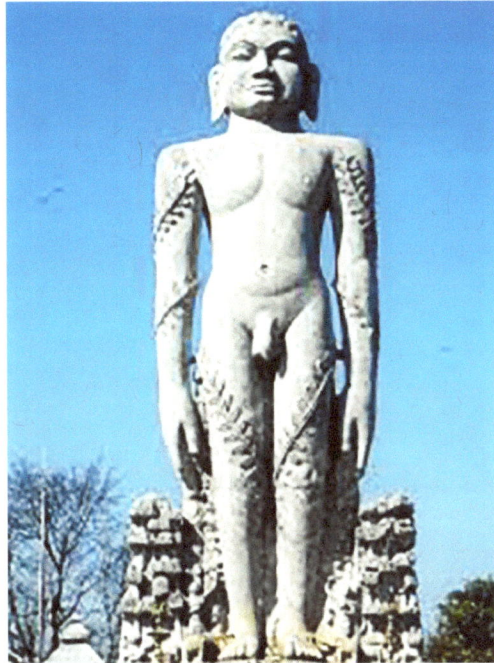

The Statue of Baahoobali (India)
A prince who later became Yogi and Monk.
He had a perfect posture, or perfectly symmetric body.

Good Posture, technically, *(in the anatomical position)* **is one when:**

1. The Center of Gravity is located at the center of the front part of the sacrum,
2. The right and left halves of the body are mirror image of each other,
3. The central line between front and back parts of the body passes through the cornel plane
4. The pair of joints like ankles, knees, shoulders and also Greater Trochanters (GT) and ears are located in coronal plane.

Usually this kind of perfection or ideal posture is rarely seen. Most of the human bodies are having bad posture (to different degrees.) But the good news is that Structural Body Work opens, for the most people, the doors of possibility of good posture.

3rd Principle of SBW
THE SKELETON AND FASCIA

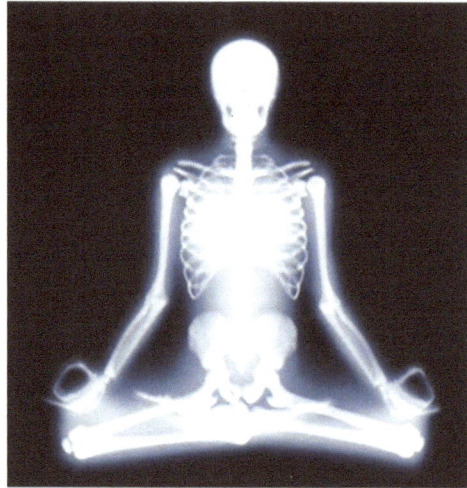

In order to understand the Structural Body Work, it is also important to know about the Fascia and its relation to the Skeleton.

Fascia is a network of fibers spread from skin to bones. It is an all-pervading flexible net of white fibers. It is the fibrous connective tissue which holds everything in the body (from skin to bones and the organs in between) together and holds them in place. There are two kind of fascia, the **Superficial facia,** located under the skin, and the **deeper fascia** which surrounds the muscles, organs, cells and blood vessels.

Function of Fascia: Since there is continuity in fascia, it connects all the cells of the body with each other, as well as every organ. It separates and simultaneously unites them and hold them in their place within the body. Fascia being elastic in its nature it helps the organs to stay in their proper place. Every cell and organ is surrounded by a layer of fascia, like a 'glove'. The whole fascial system also works as a pump for the different fluids in the body. Thus, the tension in fascia causes obstruction in normal flow of blood, lymph and other fluids of the body. Fascia is also responsible for muscle tone. Tension in fascia changes muscle tone.

For better understanding of fascia, let us imagine that fascia is a bunch of wires, ropes, strips, fabrics and fine fibers, and all these working together are holding the structure, form skin to the skeleton, as one.

The skeleton is like the poles of a building which gives space within and around. In that space the fascia comes to play. It attaches across the bones and gives stability and motion. Thus, the skeleton is not immovable like a building, but moves in space. The rest of the organs (muscles, blood vessels, and different body-systems) in the space between the fascia and the skeleton, are given a definite place. Supported by fascia, every organ stays in the same place and at the same time remains connected (directly or indirectly) with every other organ.

The long strips of fascia work in coordination with each other and thus support the movement of the body. Since different strips of fascia work in coordination with each other, it is obvious that slightest injury or hardness or tension in one part of fascia affects the other parts body.

Fascia is responsible for the shape and structure of the body:

For better understanding let us imagine that we removed all the fascia from the body of a person, keeping everything else. Well, what we do see as a result? The organs and the cells of the body are support-less and the body crumbles down like a heap of sand!

Now let us imagine that we removed all the cells and organs from the body of a person, and only fascia is left. What we see as a result? The shape of the body in the form of fascia. It is so clear that we can recognize the person.

So, in SBW, we change the Fascia to change the structure, shape and posture. We improve the structure or posture of the body by changing the shape of the whole fascia. This is done by releasing tension, hardness, constriction, atrophy etc., in the muscles, fascia, and increasing space between the joints. It releases the pressure on nerves and so also releases the pains and discomforts. It helps to improves muscle tone, flexibility, range of motion; releases the obstruction in the flow of blood and lymph, thus increases the flow of life energy, or Prana or Chi, and uplifts the mood.

The Fascia, the Ground substance and the Nervous System

A gelatin like substance surrounding the fascia is called the ground substance and is it very important for healthy fascia. There is correlation between the fascia, nervous system and the ground substance. That is why all these three are affected by massage or healing touch. It is believed that the fascia is a crystalline substance, because a touch with pressure, sometimes, gives the sensation of electric- current.

4th Principle of SBW
MOVEMENT

The Gravity of earth is the foundation of the movement of the body. So, we need to understand certain terms related to the gravity and the body:

Vertical Line of Gravity in the anatomical position, is an imaginary vertical line which passes from the center of gravity of the body to the center of earth.

Line in relation to the body is a straight line, parallel to the line of gravity. When all the segments of the body are parallel to the line of gravity they are said to be in line. This line is not considered to be static, as the body is designed to expand in all directions and contract with the force of gravity.

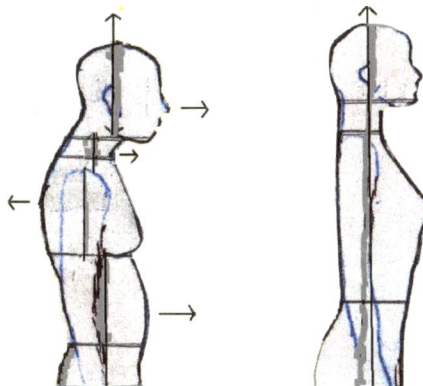

*The segments of the body on right are in the straight **"Line"***

The Vertical Line of Polarity: When the different segments of the body are in the straight line and at the same time in movement, the line is called the Line of Polarity. (The 'Line' and the 'Line of Polarity' are similar concepts)

When we lift our body with the force of gravity, this force is spread in the body in all the directions equally, through the Line of Polarity, (if the conditions are right) and this is possible with the movement called Pelvic Extension.

Pelvic Extension: When you pull your lumbar region the posterior direction, the superior part of the lumbar is extended in superior direction (towards the head) and the heels are extended in the 'inferior' direction (downwards) and L5 is pulled 'posterior', thus, the Line of Polarity extends longer. This movement is called 'Pelvic Extension'.

The Line of Polarity passes through the three rings as follows:

1-   The ring made by shoulder girdle
2-   The ring made by diaphragm
3-   The ring made by the pelvic girdle

In the ideal state of the body, these three rings are parallel to the ground and parallel to each other which help the body to be in balance, in good posture.

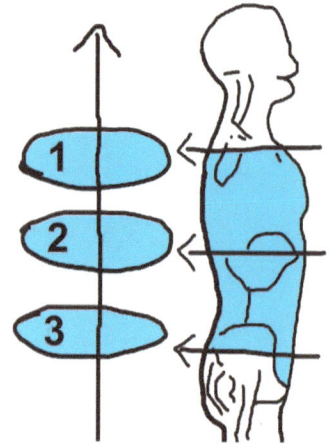

The Process of SBW

In order to bring the three rings parallel to the ground we need to remember the following points:

1. Pelvic extension helps to balance the Pelvic ring
2. The balance of the Diaphragm Ring depends on balance of Pelvic Ring
3. The balance of Shoulder Ring depends on the balance of Diaphragm ring
4. There is correlation between balance of Shoulder Ring and the Expansion of 'Horizontal Polarity' and so also the 'Upper Pole' (Head)
5. The Upper Pole has to be balanced on the Atlas (C1)

What is Horizontal line of Polarity?

Horizontal Polarity is an imaginary line parallel to the ground passing through the centers of both shoulder-joints

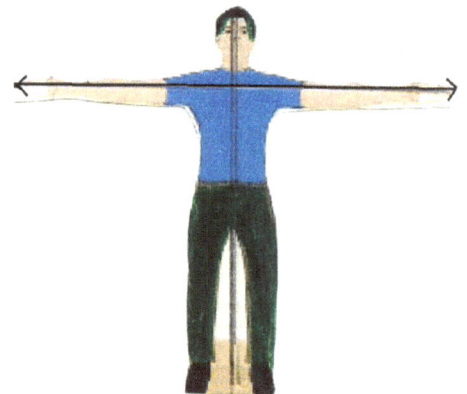

For the Expansion of horizontal line of Polarity:

The Therapist should remember: -

1. Shoulder ring must be balanced. The arms are supported by the spine through the shoulder ring, and the movements of arms are supported by the vertebral column. The arms when extended parallel to the ground are supported by mid-vertebrae. They are supported by upper vertebrae, when extended lower than shoulder joint; and are supported by lower vertebrae when extended higher than shoulder joints. Thus, the fascia of the dorsal side and the neck also must be free from tension to balance the shoulder ring first. That would help to balance the upper pole (head).

2. When the arms are extended right and left, away from the shoulder and parallel to the ground, the Horizontal Line of polarity expands., and for this purpose,

   - The shoulder joints need to be extended away from the spine, core;
   - The elbows need to be extended away from the shoulder joints and
   - The wrists need to be extended away from the elbows and so also
   - The fingers need to be extended away from the wrists.

THE UPPER POLE (HEAD)

When the head is perfectly balanced on the **Atlas, 1ˢᵗ vertebrae (C1),** the head feels like it is weightless and floating like a balloon. When the Atlas is balanced the weight of the body is distributed evenly on the two sides of the skeleton. This is possible when all the fascia of the neck is free from tension, the shoulder girdle is balanced by releasing fascia around neck and the rib cage, shoulder joints, low back etc.

Atlas, the First Vertebrae (C1)

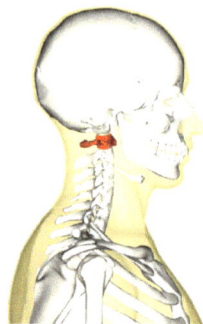

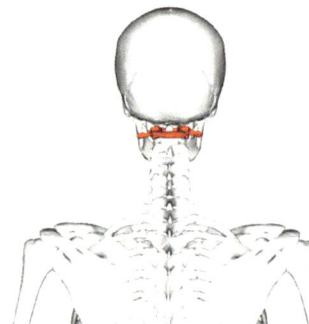

Lateral View   *Posterior View*

The anatomy of the spinal column is a precision mechanism:

The slightest shift of the Atlas from its correct anatomical location can have negative repercussions on the entire musculoskeletal, postural, circulatory and parasympathetic nervous systems, as well as the body in general. Atlas has a great influence on the balance of the spine and whole skeleton and is therefore directly responsible for an upright posture.

The Misalignment of the Atlas might be the cause of your (MSD) problems like:

Chronic pains after whiplash trauma, recurring migraine or headaches. so also functional short leg, pelvic obliquity, lordosis, kyphosis, scoliosis, loss of the cervical curvature, dizziness, unsteadiness, jaw pain, TMJD, chronic sinusitis, asthma (may have other causes) limited or painful head rotation or bending, cervical pain, stiff neck, shoulder pain – one shoulder higher, numbness of the arms, recurrent tendinitis, back pain, functional scoliosis, compressed spinal nerves, pelvic asymmetry, sacroiliac joint pain, chronically cold hands and feet, buzzing or ringing in the ears – tinnitus, hypertension, low blood pressure, depression, insomnia, chronic fatigue, allergies, Bell's Palsy, stress.

Because the Atlas supports the weight of head, about 6 pounds (which is considerable), the misaligned Atlas causes the cranium not to be perpendicular to the spine. This produces a shift in the body's center of gravity and therefore an imbalance from head to toe, leading to musculoskeletal disorder. (MDS). This causes a static false posture, in which one side of the body is more stressed than the other. As a result, pain is often concentrated on one side.

Depending on the kind of Atlas misalignment, physiological lordosis or kyphosis of the spine may intensify sharply or disappear altogether.

Therefore, it is very important for the therapist to work on the neck at the end of every session and pay specific attention towards the alignment of Atlas in the 7th session.

EXPANSIONAL BALANCE

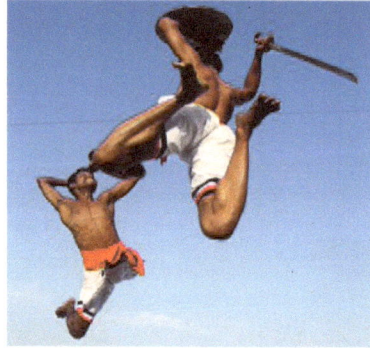

The body is said to be in expansional balance, "When the body uses the force to lift itself in the field of gravity, and the force is equally distributed through the whole body, producing one equal tensional field of force which expands the body omnidirectional in space, and it is the result of balanced polarization of two forces, one vertical and the other horizontal."

—Michel N.

The expansional balance is a key, if we may say so, to maintain the perfect body posture. Because it could be achieved when a physical culture (like Yoga, classic dance, martial art, or sports) becomes a hobby or part of life. If you are not in good shape, and are planning to start vigorous physical disciple, or an exercise program, it is good idea to get the SBW first.

Unfortunately, most people, in our modern time, are living in "Contracted" and "imbalance" rather than expansional balance. In other words, their movement against the gravity is limited. (due to variety of reasons including lack of physical discipline)

Further, there is misconception about exercise, posture etc. Even some athletes working in gym or doing sports without having the idea of 'balance', end up with hardening of the superficial layers of muscles, and disorganizing the deeper layer, losing contact with the deeper physical awareness or consciousness. Under such circumstances, SBW is the best way to regain the natural balance and deeper physical awareness.

Expansional Balance of the Therapist:

It is of vital importance for the therapist to keep himself balanced, without which, he will have hard time with his body and also difficulty helping his client. *"You cannot give what you do not have"* When you as a therapist know by experience in your body, what 'balance' is, then you will be able to help your client.

It is important to note that the therapist, does not claim to "cure" any disease. He does not impose the "heard or said" matter or principles on the body of his client. But knowing by 'experience' of his own 'balance' and knowing client's body *by perception through his hands,* he helps the client's body to open itself to the best possibilities, and put the body in the contact with the body's inner power of self-healing. That is what make a therapist a healer.

5th Principle of SBW
TOUCH AND AWARENESS

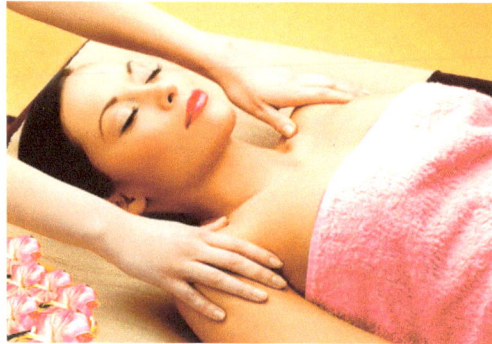

"Listen to your body's voice, the body has its own wisdom."

"The Body has a consciousness that's quite personal to it and altogether independent of mind. The body is aware of its own functioning, or its own equilibrium or disequilibrium, and it becomes absolutely conscious, in quite a precise way; If there is a disorder somewhere, it is in contact with that and feels it very clearly, even if there are no external symptoms. The body is aware of its whole working, it is harmonious, well balanced, quite regular, functioning as it should... it has that kind of plentitude... of joy... joy of living, moving in equilibrium, full of life and energy."

—(The Mother)

The vital functions of the body (heartbeat, breathing, digestion etc.) are governed by Autonomous Nervous System; (a part of Chitta), or the body consciousness, of which your mind is not aware. But it is possible for your mind to be aware of the deeper physical consciousness, if you want. Even if you choose to be unaware of what is going within, everything will continue to function, just the same, until something goes wrong and begins to manifest itself as a kind of pain or discomfort or disease, which will force you to be aware of it. You might have heard people saying, *"This problem started all of sudden, I was fine yesterday"* But in reality, the cause of the problem had started behind the veil a long time ago, and your mind, or external consciousness was unaware of it. If you were aware you could have prevented it. *SBW can help you to be aware of your body consciousness* by means of 'the communication by touch'

The communication by touch means that the therapist does not touch the body of the client but the 'body consciousness'; there upon the 'Body Consciousness' response and begins to participate in the process. Thus, the therapist helps the client to be aware of his deeper 'Body Consciousness'. In this way, the job of the therapist as well as the client becomes easier. This is a subtle process in SBW and it is called "The Communication by touch" It means the communication between the "body" (of the client) and the Body Worker (the therapist). In this way, the therapist gets information on the inner conditions of the body and how it is malfunctioning.

The process of 'communication by touch' could be summarized as follows:

Touch → sensation in the body → information to the therapist → adjust pressure accordingly → sensation → Info → adjust vector accordingly → sensation-info → further guide →

First, the therapist touches the body consciously and softly, with very minute attention, the therapist hands have "eyes" and "ears" which see and hear what is happening under the skin. Then apply pressure increasing gradually, go deeper until you feel the resistance, then choose the vector as may be necessary, and move very slowly without forcing, follow the movement of opening of the soft tissue in the body, and give passive movement to the joints, to move them away from each other, creating space between them.

During this process, the therapist may get information about conditions like type of muscle tone, knots, resistance, dryness, contraction of muscle/fascia, and the subtle sensations and reactions of the body.

When the therapist becomes aware of the sensations of the client's body, the client also, at the same time becomes aware of it, (provided the client is focused and paying attention to the touch.) With experience, the therapist may sometimes get an intuitive knowledge of the problematic area of the body.

2 | THE THEORY

THE NECESSARY CONDITIONS FOR 'THE COMMUNICATION BY TOUCH'

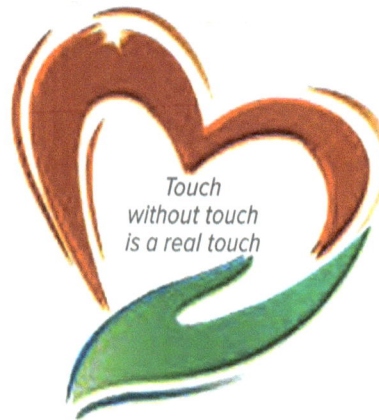

Touch
without touch
is a real touch

1. The therapist must touch the 'Consciousness of the Body'
2. The therapist as well as the client must be focused.
3. The atmosphere around should be free from disturbances
4. Preferably no presence of third person in the room.
5. The client/ patient /health aspirant must be instructed as follows:

Instructions to the client /patient/ health aspirant:

1. **'Pay attention to my touch.'** This is primary requirement. The client is not allowed to let his mind wander.

2. **'Let the energy of my hands enter into your body.'** In other words, the client has to be receptive and receptive means, 'Leave the muscles loose when touched by the therapist and absorb the energy from the hands of therapist into his own body. With this understanding the receptivity increases.

3. **'Pay attention to all the physical sensations arising in your body'** (by touch) When the client pays attention to the sensations, his interest in inner experience increases, and he becomes aware of the 'Deeper Physical Consciousness, which knows how to heal the body.

4. **'Use my hands'.** When the client has reached the stage 3 as above, and his Deeper Physical Consciousness actively participates in the process of healing, by using your art of touch, your energy, your knowledge behind the touch, then often his Physical or Body consciousness drags your hands to the part of his body where it is necessary to do some special work, and you receive the guidance for the next step.

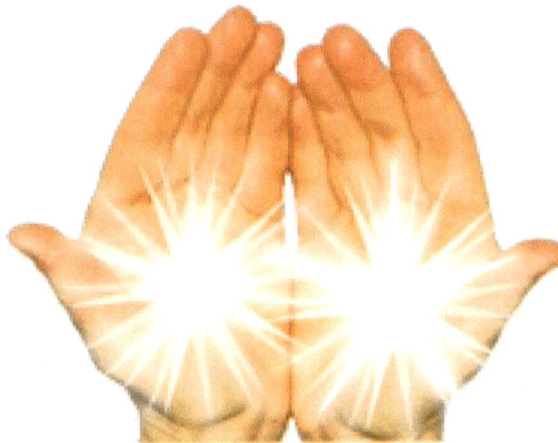

THE THEMES OF STRUCTURAL BODY WORK

'The Structural Body Work' is a series of ten sessions. Every session proceeds with a specific theme. *A specific part of the body is treated and as a result, some specific physical and psychological changes are noted.*

Important Note:

- These themes and the order of treatments are designed by Dr. Ida Rolf.
- The therapist is advised to follow the course of treatments in the same order
- If you try to change the order, it may have negative consequences
- Once you start the SBW, you must be committed to work till all ten sessions are completed.
- The client must be informed that if he decides to stop the SBW, he may do so before the 4th session. If he decides to continue thereafter, he must be committed to finish the rest of all sessions; failing to do so, may have negative consequences on his body.

It is important to know the message of each theme, and how it relates to the work done in the corresponding session; the work which brings about the physical changes followed by the possible psychological changes.

UNDERSTANDING THE THEMES OF SBW

Physically, Emotionally, Anatomically,
Materially, Psychologically & Spiritually

Session 1. *The Theme: 'Inspiration'*

Inspiration means 'breathing' and to be inspired'. There is a close relationship between the two. The pattern of breathing and the psychological state are related to each other. You might have noticed that your breathing pattern changes according to your emotions like anger, peace, love, happiness excitement, depression, or relaxation, concentration and meditation. The Pranayama, an aspect of Hatha Yoga, is based on this fact of close connection between the psychological state and the breathing pattern.

Further, the Pranayama or inspiration is not just deep breathing, but to draw the 'Prana' or 'Chi' or Life energy from the Universe and to get in touch of the inner spirit and be inspired. *(You may try this: At times, when it is difficult to make right decision, try not think hard, instead, sit down quietly in a corner, and do slow and deep breathing, focusing on the top of your head, sooner or later you might be inspired, and know what is the right decision)*

The respiratory system is the foundation of breathing and life. If the organs, muscles and fascia related to the respiratory system are tense or restricted, your breathing power is limited, and it has negative consequences on physical and psychological health.

In the first session of SBW, we focus the on the organs, or muscles-fascia directly or indirectly related to your respiratory system in order to release the tension and restrictions, so that you can breathe better, feel energetic and relaxed.

Session 2. *The Theme: 'Standing on your own feet'* or to be independent

To be independent does not mean 'not to accept support from any one'. You need support of earth to stand on your feet. Your feet will be useless if there is no

53

2 | THE THEORY

ground. But the earth will not help you, if your feet are weak or unsteady. Thus, it is the matter of a balance between dependence and independence.

Anatomically: In this session, we work on the muscle-fascia, ligaments, and tendons related to your feet and try to release the tension in those areas to bring your feet in balance.

Session 3. *The Theme: 'Reaching out'*

Reaching out means to reach others to receive and offer any help, to expand the areas of contact; to embrace, to be kind, compassionate, loving.

It also means to protect oneself and the others from the violence, to fight for the cause of truth. In all the actions as stated above we use our arms. The word 'arms' is also used for the weapons we use for fighting or protecting. But to do so we also need strong and balanced arms, and therefore the balanced between reasoning and emotions.

Anatomically, we focus, in third session, on the muscles- fascia related to your arms, and release limitation constriction, tension in those areas.

Session 4. *The Theme: 'Control and Surrender'*

The first control we learn in life is to control the urge to urinate and defecate, (the organ located in pelvic region), to be able to do in a right place. Control means to hold and surrender mean to give up, let go. Control does not necessarily mean to have hardness, oppression, rigidity, tyranny. Healthy control is sentimental, delicate and creative.

Surrender does not mean weakness; True surrender is the surrender of the ego. *('Ishvar Pranidhaan' as in Yoga Sutra)'* In surrender there is confidence in relations, it is free from the worry of the future, it has faith in divine grace. It is possible to have both, control and the surrender simultaneously. It is a question of balance between control and surrender.

Anatomically, we focus on the muscles-fascia of the part of the body that are related to the pelvic floor which influences the flow of energies in the organs located in pelvic floor. It also helps to balance the sense of control and surrender.

Session 5. *The Theme: 'Guts'*

By the Guts we mean courage. It also indicates digestive organs; and it is true that the state of your organs related to digestive system, and your feeling of courage or fear are related to each other.

The first thing that goes in our gut is the mother's milk, which gives the nourishment, love, sense of security and also courage. In India there is a proverb, used in challenging situations, *"Have you had your mother's milks?"*

It is simply to say if you have any courage.

It is important to note that

- A sudden sensation of fear is experienced in guts, around the naval region.
- The guts, the digestive system transforms the energy from food into life energy
- We prefer to have meals with those we love.
- Our psychological states effect the guts, digestive systems.
- Emotional Trauma has negative impact on belly region, specifically psoas, Abs, Diaphragm
- Eating disorders are often related to some psychological or emotional disturbances.

Anatomically, in the 5th session, we work to release the tension or imbalance in your guts or the organs or muscle- fascia related, directly or indirectly, to your digestive system, also releasing emotional trauma, if any.

Session 6. *The theme: 'Holding Back'*

Emotionally: It means holding negative memories of the past, keep regretting, and preventing the self from creative work or moving ahead to a better future.

Materially: It means to be disorganized, hoarder, greedy.

Both of the above are related to each other.

Anatomically, in this session, we try to release the tension and disorder in the dorsal side of your body, specifically the muscles fascia of the posterior legs, consequently releasing tension form the past.

Session 7. *The theme: 'Lose your head'*

Physically, it means 'to free the neck from tension so that you have the free movement of the head, (the skull and Atlas)

Emotionally, it means to be free from mental stress, self-centered thought, and useless thinking. Both of the above are related to each other. 'thinking' and intelligence is a very important part of your personality, but most of the time, the activities in your brain are only the mechanical and uncontrolled movements, which is tiresome. They have nothing to do with the intelligence. We are not, most of the time, aware of the ceaseless activities going on within our brain.

Anatomically, in the 7th session, we organize the muscle-fascia of the neck and release it from tension and balance the head over neck or Alas; consequently, it helps to balance the reasoning and emotions, and so the head feels weightless and free from tension.

Session 8. *The Theme: 'Feminine Aspect'*

The part of the body, from naval and pelvic region (*related to Manipur and Swadhisthan Chakra)* to feet, is a symbol of femininity. Your body is part of your mother's body, and it is connected with this part (below naval) of her body. Your feet are connected to the Mother Earth. *(Biologically, 'The Mitochondria is received only from the mother's genes)*

The femininity is the name of Energy (*Shakti*), Beauty and Prosperity (*Laxmi*). It is manifested in your personality, not only by exterior beauty and form, but by the inner Energy and the Receptivity.

Note that every man has, in himself, a feminine aspect, too. (Ya devi sarva bhuteshu Matri rupen samsthita...The Mother that dwells in all beings...)

In this session, the part of the body related to the feminine aspect is released from tension, helping you to have balance between the feminine and masculine aspects of your personality.

Session 9. *The Theme: 'Masculine Aspect'*

The upper part of your body, (arms, shoulders, chest) *is* the symbol of the masculine aspect, the symbol of action, success and to initiate action. In the modern life, we insist on the masculine aspect, but forget that we can attain the success only by 'balancing the masculine and feminine aspects of our personality.

Anatomically, in this session, we work on the part of your body related to the masculine aspect of your personality to balance it with the feminine aspect.

Session 10: *The theme 'Integration and Perfection'*

Physically, integration means organization and coordination of all parts of your body, like an orchestra playing music.

Psychologically, to have balance between your mind and emotions, having no contradictions among different parts of your being *and*

Spiritually, to find your true self, to know oneself, or the deeper self which knows how to be happy, healthy and joyful.

In the 10th session we try to integrate and harmonize all parts of your body and open the doors of health and happiness that is already within you. Nothing is added from outside.

MYSTERIOUS EXPERIENCES

Structural Body Work (SBW) & Neuro-Spinal Analysis (NSA)

(From Notes: 09/15/08)

The information given here may give you better vision of SBW

Due to recent low back injury, there was some structural deformation pain and stiffness. As a result, my mind was, at times, foggy, or suddenly felt like vegetating. I went to Neha Curtis, my teacher of Structural Work.

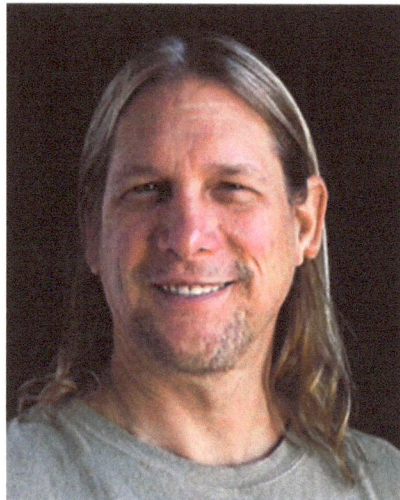

Neha Curtiss,
Director, Healing Hands School of Holistic Health, Escondido, CA USA

During the second session of SBW with Neha, I had mysterious experience while he was working on my left foot:

My mind was completely relaxed, almost like in the state of meditation, yet it was different, in a sense that my mind was mysteriously connected to my foot and the connection was NOT via flesh or bone or fascia or anything material. There was deep peace in the head and at the same time there was a kind of deep pain in the foot. But it did not bother me. The experience was completely different than our normal physical mental experience. It was a wonderful state of being (I wish I could live in that state all the time)

Two hours later, when I had gone back home, I felt my shoulder girdle suddenly unwounded (it was twisted before) and my body seemed more balanced. Later in 15 minutes, I became aware in my physical consciousness that I was holding lots of tension on my facial muscles (after the injury), as I became aware, the fascial tension was released all of sudden.

That afternoon, I had an appointment with Dr. Whelan, D.C. (Laguna Hills) At his work place, there were several patients in ventral position on different massage tables. While I was waiting my turn, I witnessed amazing performance of Dr. Whalen.

For example:

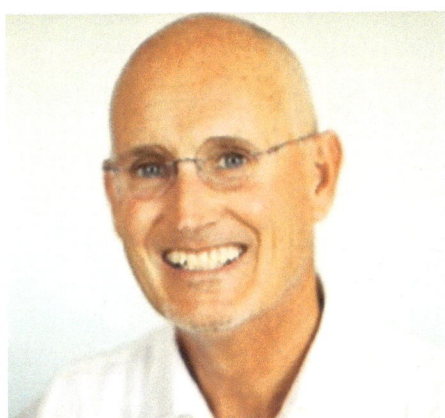

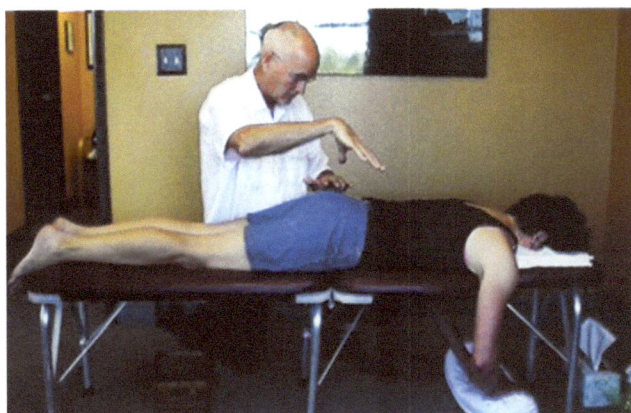

Dr. Whelan D. C. Laguna Hills, CA USA

Dr. Whalen held his palm in space over spine of a patient and the body of the patient began to vibrate strongly. He did some gesture of sewing with an invisible needle and thread, above the spine and the body began some strange movements. He placed his fist over a table near the waist of a client without touching the client and twisted the wrist; and the body of the client began to twist. It looked like magic.

I was curious to know how it worked. I asked him if he would not mind explaining it to me. He was very kind intelligent and humble. It was a joyful event to have conversation with him. He let me watch his work for a while then he would call me near some patients and would ask me, "Where you think the Chi (Prana) is blocked?" I would look at the body and then would point out some area of the body. *"Right" he said, "Watch now"*, and then he would do something over the area I pointed out and the body would begin to move.

He also tried to explain the theory.

What I understood from his explanation was thus:

- A Structural Body Worker or Rolfer (like Neha) changes the structure of the body, and it results into the change in Consciousness or Awareness.
- Dr. Whelan worked to bring the change in Awareness or Consciousness and it resulted into the change in Structure of the body.

Conclusion:

Both, Neha and Dr. Whalen worked with the same principle but from two opposite poles, and they both meet at the same central point (the healthy state) which Neha calls *"A State of health being constantly Enhancing"* and Dr Whalen called it as *"Turn back on the path of evolution."* And for me it is one and the same thing namely, *"A progressive balance between body mind and spirit"*

In brief the formula is:

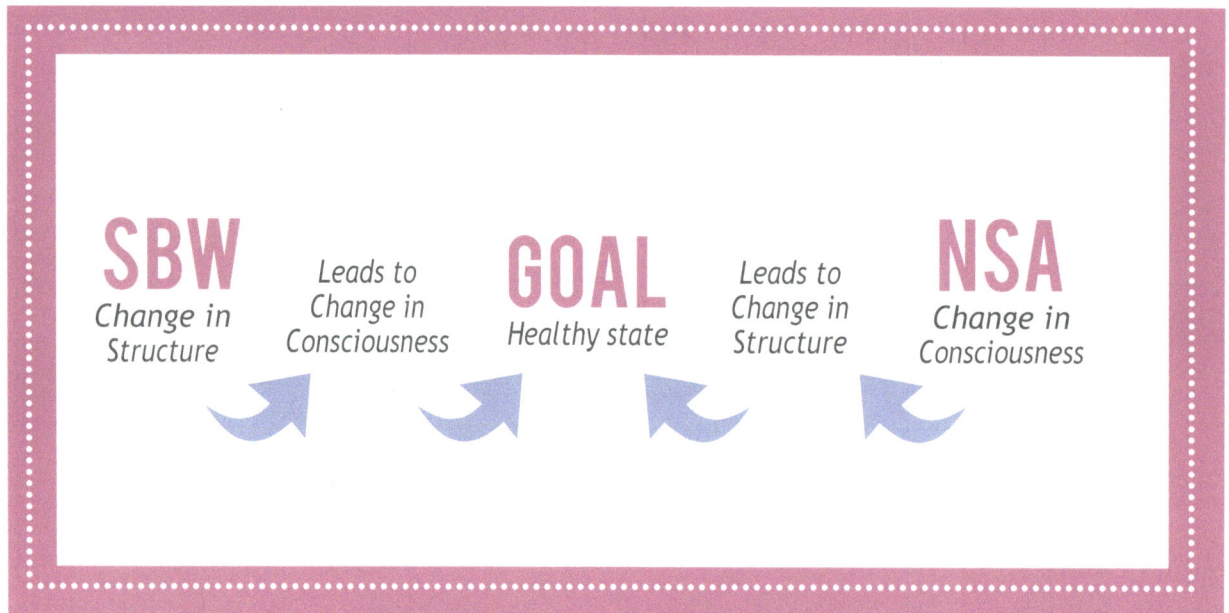

SBW
Change in Structure

Leads to Change in Consciousness

GOAL
Healthy state

Leads to Change in Structure

NSA
Change in Consciousness

I was inspired. I had a flash. "Is it possible to combine SBW and NSA?"

Why not? If we can get the secret key, that Dr Whelan has, to manipulate Prana or Chi, then the central goal, the healthy state, (which we defined in three different ways as above) could be attained with less time and less effort. The reason I say so is that, SBW requires less time but more physical efforts on the

60

part of therapist as well as the patient; while NSA requires hardly any effort but it takes longer time comparatively. So, if we can combine SBW and NSA we could have best result in less time without much effort.

Back to Dr. Whalen's office:

It was my turn now. I was on the table in ventral position. Whalen did touch my back very lightly, but to my surprise, my body did not respond. The reason he said was that I had lots of input and my energy gates were not sensitized. I did not know what he meant but then he told, "Because you have lots of 'Chi" (Prana Shakti).

Dr. Whalen had taken picture of my body profile 'two days' ago. It indicated that my neck was inclined up to 10 degrees. He took another picture of my profile then. And he saw there was no inclination at all. And he was surprised, he had an unforgettable joyful healthy big laugh; *"I have never seen such thing in my life."* He said.

After 3rd session with Neha on 9/29/08, I visited Dr. Whelan again. He did something over my body but my body did not respond.

Anyway, Dr. Whalen looked at my body posture carefully again and he said with a surprise, *"The body looks almost normal, only after 3 treatments of SBW, and so much improvement, so much energized?* And thus, he became very curious about the Structural Work and Neha. *"I would like to meet the man (Neha) who is working on you" he said.*

"Can you ask Neha to come to my office?" He asked. But both of them, Neha and Dr. Whelan had very busy schedule. I could not arrange their meeting.

**However, it is still a matter of research
'How to manipulate Prana/Chi; and combine the two therapies namely, Structural Body work and Neuro-Spinal Analysis?'**

UNDERSTANDING HOLISTIC THERAPIES
(Tips for Holistic Health Practitioners and Health Aspirants)

There are variety of Holistic and Alternative Therapies in the world. Each of them is good in its own place. Each works for some kind of ailments but not for all.

It is possible that a patient has tried all possible medical treatments and yet did not get better. Maybe the diagnosis of the disease was inaccurate, or the cause of the disease was not only physical but also emotional or psychological. So, one must look for inner causes of the illness.

According to the Mother, a disease is always an outer expression of inner disharmony. One must look for the inner cause of the disease rather than the outer. ***The cause of disease is certainly a loss of equilibrium within.*** Disequilibrium are of many kinds for example:

Physical disequilibrium or imbalance:

When all the organs of the body are working in coordination with one another, there is no pain or disease. But if something goes wrong with any part of the body, the whole body may go wrong, more or less seriously or even an accident may happen.

Physical disequilibrium is of two kinds, **Structural and functional**

1. Structural Disequilibrium (subject of SBW)

- Disequilibrium due to inner cause or
- Disequilibrium due to outer cause or environment or accident, injury.

Understanding Structural Disequilibrium:

When any organ is injured or tense, then suddenly or gradually the whole body may fall sick, to lesser or greater extent. For example, an injury in muscle or ligament or any organ caused by an accident may gradually develop into serious disease, pain, discomfort or disintegration; and it is difficult to regain the equilibrium. Here the SBW is the best solution.

2. Functional Disequilibrium

- The cause of disequilibrium could be within
- The cause of Disequilibrium could be outer/ environmental

Understanding Functional Disequilibrium

- When one of the organs refuses to cooperate with rest, e.g. heart is suddenly pumping very fast. In such case you may control the heart by Pranayama.

- When there is quarrel or arguments within. For example, your body wants to rest and at the same time your mind wants to work. What will you do? Listen to your mind or body? Then at the same time if your emotional being in revolt, the inner quarrel could be severe and you fall very sick. Further, if there is also mental disequilibrium which could be a kind of confusion, worry, anxiety, then your condition could get worst. You can imagine number of diverse causes of inner disequilibrium and diseases.

- When the structural and/or functional imbalance (due to inner or outer cause) is compounded by an emotional issue like fear, disappointment, guilt etc. that is followed by mental disequilibrium (negative thinking or negative suggestion form environment), then a simple issue like headache or back pain can end up becoming an apparently incurable disease. No therapy works.

In such cases, one may want to understand the psychology of the patient, make him reflect on his inner conflict. Suggest him to try the cleansing process of Hatha Yoga, Naturopathy, healthy diet, Pranayama etc. That would certainly help, along with appropriate other treatment depending on the symptoms.

FACTORS IN HEALING

The Force, Instrument, Instrumentation and Receptivity

Most body workers, especially healers, know that ultimately it is the Force (Cosmic Energy, Shakti, Prana, Chi, or name anything you like) that helps the healing. The therapist is the Instrument through whom the Force works and the technique used by therapist is the Instrumentation.

In rare occasions, the therapists may come across some clients who wish (deep in their heart) **not** to be cured, because they think they are loved or cared or paid special attention only when they are sick. (sometimes they express it verbally) It is hard or almost impossible to help them. And even if they are cured somehow, sooner or later they fall sick again.

This means that the receptivity and willingness of the client is also necessary in a healing process.

Further the extent of receptivity of the client depends on his conscious cooperation, (presence of mind) and so also on the state of his body. Thus, the body that is exercised or disciplined in some way is more receptive than one who is lethargic, or one who has neglected to pay attention to their physical issues or do anything about it unless when absolutely necessary.

Leading spirit of the client as well as the trust in the hands therapist also increases his receptivity.

THE SOURCE OF HOLISTIC THERAPIES

Dr. Sunil Joshi, (Mrityunjaya Mission, Ayurveda Institute, Haridwar, India) has been doing research on the subject for over 25 years. He has published many books. The information found in one of his books, is summarized as follows:

Branches of Holistic Medicine from Veda

(Hindu Scripture more than 10,000 BC)

ATHARVANI	ANGIRASI	DAIVI	MANUSHI	OTHER
SPIRITUAL HEALING BY POWER OF INTENTION, WILL *(Includes Pranic Healing, Reiki, Nyas or Visualization Self Hypnosis)*	**MARMA THERAPY:** Healing by stimulating secretions or chemicals in the body by touching, pressing, rubbing or punching at the specific points on the body *(Includes Acupressure, Acupuncture, Reflexology, Dry Massages, Skin rolling)*	**TREATMENT WITH NATURAL ELEMENTS:** Mud, water, air, solar light, space • Eight-fold Ayurveda • Medicine • Surgery • Toxicology • Psychology • Pediatrics • Aphrodisiac+ *(Includes checking pulse & other vibrations in the body, Herbal Oil Massages Potali etc.)*	• **Different types of medicines invented by men** • **Eight-fold Yoga** • **Hatha Yoga** *(Includes number of cleansing processes, Asanas, Pranayama Pratyahara Concentration Meditation and more)*	• **Asuri** Violent treatments, Like burning certain points on skin by hot iron rod, Cupping, etc. • **Madhuvidya** • **Pragvidya** • **Mrita-sanjivani-vidya** (science of resuscitation) *Some of these have been lost with time*

The source of Holistic Therapies continue...

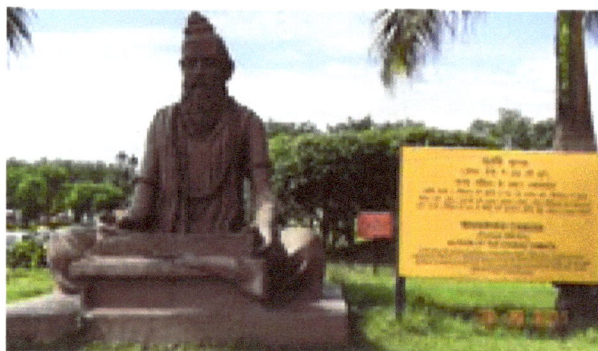

Maharshi Charak

A few of the therapies from **'Charak Samhita'** *written by a great Physician and Yogi Charak, 200 BC, are as follows:*

DIAVYA VYAPASHRAYA	YUKTI VYAPASHRAYA	SATVAJAYA
Crystals, Mantra, Mala, Rudraksha and Tulsi beads Pranayama, fasting, Pranipat	Appropriate foods Appropriate activates Herbal Medicine	Spiritual means Yoga Surrender to the Supreme

YOGA and SBW

Yoga is a Psychological Process. It is Change in (or upward movement of) our Consciousnesses, gradually from normal to super-normal, at different levels of our Being (physical, mental, emotional, and deeper layers of our existence) and changing our approach or understanding of life and one self, which brings the Joy in life independent of external conditions of life. The side effects of physical aspect of yoga (i.e. Hatha Yoga including meditation) are good posture, lasting health, "Slim body and Brightness".

What we call yoga in popular term, is limited to Asanas, or stretching, a kind of exercise, related to physical aspect only; yet, if practiced correctly, improves posture and health, makes you aware of deep physical consciousness, and uplifts mental, emotional states, too.

SWB starts dealing with our physical aspect, and helps to improve body- posture, there by releasing pain patterns, helps to be aware of deeper physical consciousness and uplifting mental, emotional state.

COMPARE THE PROCESS OF SBW AND HATHA YOGA

SBW: PROCESS & BENEFITS (Minimum of 10 Sessions)	YOGA: PROCESS &BENEFITS Few of the Corresponding Asanas etc. in Yoga with same & more Benefits
Session: 1. Inspiration: Rib-cage and body parts related to respiratory system are being made free from tension.	**Pranayama** done in right way is the most powerful way to make your respiratory system stronger. It also awakes the deeper physical awareness. It helps to tap into cosmic Energy that is more effective.
Session 2. Standing on your own feet: It helps to release constriction in feet and legs	**Asanas:** Padangushth-, (making toes, soles Achilleas, calves supple) Utkatra, Makara, Supta-Vajra-
Session: 3. Reaching out: The muscle fascia of the arms and torso become flexible	**Asana as:** Ushta-, Shalabha-, Bhujanga-, Gomikha-, Trikon-, Tada-, Ardha-matsyendra-
Session 4. Control and surrender: Bring flexibility in the muscle-fascia of medial legs	**Asanas:** Butterfly, Bhadra, Matsya, Padma-
Session 5. Guts (digestive): Releases any tension in organs/fascia related to digestive system, thereby releases emotional trauma	**Asanas:** Mayur, Manduka, Kurma, Matsya,Ushtra, Chakra- , **Mudra:** Tadagi **Other:** Bhastrika, Kapal-Bhati, Agnisar, Nauli
Session 6. Holding back: Posterior part of the body is made free from tension; emotionally free from negative dormant memories of past.	**Asanas** Pashchimosttan, Janushir, Ardha-Matyendra, Markata... Padangushtha-(affecting also pelvic floor and obturator internus along with posterior distal legs)
Session 7. Lose your head: Releases any tension, stiffness, stress in neck, facial muscles, mouth cavity, nasal cavities.	**Asanas:** Sarvanga, Kandhara-; **Bandh:** Jalandhar **Mudras:** Brahma-, Simha-, Khechari- **Other:** Sutra-Neti, Jal-Neti; **Dhauti:** Danta, Karna- **Pranayama:** Ujjayi, Bhramari
Sessions 8, 9, 10. Integrate all of the above	Correspond to all of above.
Most of you can benefit from SBW	**Any of you can benefit from Yoga unless** you have a serious, painful MSD. In such case you may need SBW.
Result of SBW makes your body pain free, supple, more capable and conscious and allows you to practice Yoga easily.	**Result** of discipline of daily Yoga practices keep yvour body healthy & youthful, more supple, capable and conscious and allows you to enjoy your life much better.

2/15/19

Dear Nina

     I Think your book
is well thought out &
organized...

     My best to you,
you Healer...

Paula

Healing Hands School of Holisic Health
Escondido, California, USA

9 781646 200122